Workforce and Diversity in Psychiatry

Editors

HOWARD Y. LIU
ALTHA J. STEWART

CHILD AND ADOLESCENT PSYCHIATRIC CLINICS OF NORTH AMERICA

www.childpsych.theclinics.com

Consulting Editor
JUSTINE LARSON

January 2024 • Volume 33 • Number 1

ELSEVIER

1600 John F. Kennedy Boulevard • Suite 1800 • Philadelphia, Pennsylvania, 19103-2899

http://www.theclinics.com

CHILD AND ADOLESCENT PSYCHIATRIC CLINICS OF NORTH AMERICA Volume 33, Number 1
January 2024 ISSN 1056–4993, ISBN-13: 978-0-443-12891-2

Editor: Megan Ashdown
Developmental Editor: Shivank Joshi

Child and Adolescent Psychiatric Clinics of North America (ISSN 1056-4993) is published quarterly by Elsevier Inc., 360 Park Avenue South, New York, NY 10010-1710. Months of issue are January, April, July, and October. Business and Editorial Offices: 1600 John F. Kennedy Boulevard, Suite 1800, Philadelphia, PA 19103-2899. Periodicals postage paid at New York, NY and additional mailing offices. Subscription prices are $373.00 per year (US individuals), $100.00 per year (US & Canadian students), $424.00 per year (Canadian individuals), $487.00 per year (international individuals), and $200.00 per year (international students). For institutional access pricing please contact Customer Service via the contact information below. International air speed delivery is included in all *Clinics* subscription prices. All prices are subject to change without notice. **POSTMASTER:** Send address changes to *Child and Adolescent Psychiatric Clinics of North America*, Elsevier Health Sciences Division, Subscription Customer Service, 3251 Riverport Lane, Maryland Heights, MO 63043. **Customer Service: 1-800-654-2452 (U.S. and Canada); 314-447-8871 (outside U.S. and Canada). Fax: 314-447-8029. E-mail:** JournalsCustomerService-usa@elsevier.com **(for print support) or** journalsonlinesupport-usa@elsevier.com **(for online support).**

Reprints. For copies of 100 or more of articles in this publication, please contact the Commercial Reprints Department, Elsevier Inc., 360 Park Avenue South, New York, New York 10010-1710 Tel.: 212-633-3874; Fax: 212-633-3820, E-mail: reprints@elsevier.com.

Child and Adolescent Psychiatric Clinics of North America is covered in *MEDLINE/PubMed (Index Medicus), ISI, SSCI, Research Alert, Social Search, Current Contents,* and *EMBASE/Excerpta Medica.*

Contributors

CONSULTING EDITOR

JUSTINE LARSON, MD, MPH, DFAACAP
Medical Director, Schools and Residential Treatment, Consulting Editor, Child and Adolescent Psychiatric Clinics of North America, Sheppard Pratt, Rockville, Maryland, USA

EDITORS

HOWARD Y. LIU, MD, MBA
Chair and Professor, Department of Psychiatry, University of Nebraska Medical Center, Omaha, Nebraska, USA

ALTHA J. STEWART, MD
Senior Associate Dean for Community Health Engagement, Associate Professor and Director, Division of Public and Community Psychiatry, Director, Center for Health in Justice Involved Youth, 145th President, American Psychiatric Association (2018-2019), University of Tennessee Health Science Center, Memphis, Tennessee, USA

AUTHORS

EMILY ADAMS, MS
Behavioral Health Education Center of Nebraska, University of Nebraska Medical Center, Omaha, Nebraska, USA

JEAN-MARIE E. ALVES-BRADFORD, MD
Associate Clinical Professor, Columbia University, Department of Psychiatry, New York, New York, USA

SHELLI AVENEVOLI, PhD
Deputy Director, National Institute of Mental Health, National Institutes of Health, Bethesda, Maryland, USA

MOGENS BILL BAERENTZEN, PhD, CRC, LMHP
Project Coordinator, Mid-America Mental Health Technology Transfer Center, University of Nebraska Medical Center, Omaha, Nebraska, USA

TAMI D. BENTON, MD
Psychiatrist-in-Chief, Executive Director and Chair, Department of Child and Adolescent Psychiatry and Behavioral Sciences, Children's Hospital of Philadelphia, HUB e Center for Clinical Collaboration, Philadelphia, Pennsylvania, USA

TASHALEE R. BROWN, MD, PhD
SAMHSA Minority Fellow and AACAP's Diversity, Equity, and Inclusion (DEI) Emerging Leaders Fellow, University of California Los Angeles, California, USA

QUINN CAPERS IV, MD
Rody P. Cox Professor of Medicine (Cardiology), Department of Medicine, The University of Texas Southwestern Medical Center, Dallas, Texas, USA

CRYSTAL T. CLARK, MD, MSc
Associate Professor, Department of Psychiatry, University of Toronto, Associate Head of Research, Department of Psychiatry, Women's College Hospital, Scientist, Women's College Hospital, Toronto, Ontario, Canada

AMIRA COLLISON, MD
Resident, Department of Psychiatry and Biobehavioral Sciences, Semel Institute for Neuroscience and Human Behavior, University of California, Los Angeles, Los Angeles, California, USA

DENNIS DACARETT-GALEANO, MD, MPH
Resident, Department of Psychiatry and Biobehavioral Sciences, Semel Institute for Neuroscience and Human Behavior, University of California, Los Angeles, Los Angeles, California, USA

MARLEY DOYLE, MD
Associate Professor, Behavioral Health Education Center of Nebraska, University of Nebraska Medical Center, Omaha, Nebraska, USA

ANNE D. EMMERICH, MD
Psychiatrist, Massachusetts General Hospital Department of Psychiatry, Boston, Massachusetts, USA

LAURA E. FLORES, PhD
University of Nebraska Medical Center, Omaha, Nebraska, USA

MAMTA GAUTAM, MD, MBA
Associate Professor, Psychosocial Oncology, Cancer Center, The Ottawa Hospital, Ottawa, Canada

JOSHUA A. GORDON, MD, PhD
Director, National Institute of Mental Health, National Institutes of Health, Bethesda, Maryland, USA

ALLISON GRENNAN, PhD
Assistant Professor, Department of Psychology, Munroe-Meyer Institute for Genetics and Rehabilitation, Omaha, Nebraska, USA

LAUREN D. HILL, PhD
Acting Director, Office for Disparities Research and Workforce Diversity, National Institute of Mental Health, National Institutes of Health, Bethesda, Maryland, USA

ASALE HUBBARD, PhD
Assistant Professor, University of California, San Francisco Department of Psychiatry and Behavioral Sciences, Weill Institute for Neurosciences, San Francisco VA Medical Center, San Francisco, California, USA

WARREN YIU KEE NG, MD, MPH
Medical Director, Outpatient Behavioral Health and Director of Clinical Services for the Division of Child and Adolescent Psychiatry, Columbia University Irving Medical Center, New York-Presbyterian Hospital, Morgan Stanley Children's Hospital, New York, USA

ALLISON R. LARSON, MD, MS
Academic Chair for Dermatology, Georgetown University Medical Center, MedStar Health, Washington, DC, USA

HOWARD Y. LIU, MD, MBA
Chair and Professor, Department of Psychiatry, University of Nebraska Medical Center, Omaha, Nebraska, USA

CHRISTINA MANGURIAN, MD, MAS
Professor, University of California, San Francisco Department of Psychiatry and Behavioral Sciences, Weill Institute for Neurosciences, San Francisco, California, USA

MICHAEL O. MENSAH, MD, MPH
Postdoctoral Fellow, National Clinician Scholars Program, Department of Medicine, Yale School of Medicine, New Haven, Connecticut, USA

RANNA PAREKH, MD, MPH
Chief Diversity, Equity and Inclusion Officer, The University of Texas, Anderson Cancer Center, Houston, Texas, USA

JENNIFER L. PAYNE, MD
Professor and Vice Chair of Research, Department of Psychiatry and Neurobehavioral Sciences, University of Virginia, Charlottesville, Virginia, USA

UJJWAL RAMTEKKAR, MD, MBA, MPE
Adjunct Professor, Department of Psychiatry, University of Missouri School of Medicine, Columbia, Missouri, USA

JENNIFER B. REESE, PsyD
Behavioral Health Education and Training Manager, Department of Psychiatry and Behavioral Health, Nationwide Children's Hospital, Columbus, Ohio, USA

ERIN OBERMEIER SCHNEIDER, MSW
Associate Director of External Affairs, Behavioral Health Education Center of Nebraska, University of Nebraska Medical Center, Omaha, Nebraska, USA

JULIE K. SILVER, MD
Associate Chair & Associate Professor, Department of Physical Medicine & Rehabilitation, Harvard Medical School, Boston, Massachusetts, USA

ALTHA J. STEWART, MD
Senior Associate Dean for Community Health Engagement, Associate Professor and Director, Division of Public and Community Psychiatry, Director, Center for Health in Justice Involved Youth, 145th President, American Psychiatric Association (2018-2019), University of Tennessee Health Science Center, Memphis, Tennessee, USA

SHERITTA A. STRONG, MD, DFAPA
Associate Professor, University of Nebraska Medical Center, Omaha, Nebraska, USA

ANDREW SUDLER, MD, MPH
Resident, University of California, San Francisco Department of Psychiatry and Behavioral Sciences, Weill Institute for Neurosciences, San Francisco, California, USA

LIA THOMAS, MD
Professor, Department of Psychiatry, The University of Texas Southwestern Medical Center, Dallas, Texas, USA

NHI-HA TRINH, MD, MPH
Director, MGH Psychiatry Center for Diversity, Inclusion, and Belonging, Massachusetts General Hospital, Department of Psychiatry, Boston, Massachusetts, USA

SHINOBU WATANABE-GALLOWAY, PhD
Professor, Dr. Tim Hawks Chair in Cancer Prevention and Population Science, Associate Director for Buffett Cancer Center Community Outreach & Engagement, College of Public Health, University of Nebraska Medical Center, Omaha, Nebraska, USA

Contents

Long-standing challenges facing the mental health system require more effective strategies to furnish a workforce whose diversity matches an increasingly diverse population. Current and former system leaders can offer expert guidance informed by their experiences and perspectives. Their professional journeys to leadership in this area provide context and unique insight into issues of justice, including workforce diversity, equity, and inclusion in psychiatry. These experts agree that significant policy changes are needed to improve psychiatric workforce diversity and that implementing change will require that disparate groups together to achieve this goal. Financial considerations must be included in policy and advocacy.

Documented disparities have profoundly impacted the training and careers of physicians from socially and historically marginalized groups, including women, people with disabilities, people who identify with racial and ethnic minority groups, and the lesbian, gay, bisexual, transgender, and queer or questioning+ community. Professionalism is a core component of medical training and practice, yet a focus on workforce diversity, equity, and inclusion is often absent. This report aims to encourage the adoption of workforce diversity, equity, and inclusion as a crucial component of professionalism, with an emphasis on the field of psychiatry.

States all across the United States are experiencing a shortage in their behavioral health workforces. Although many studies have suggested factors that contribute to or mitigate the shortage—particularly in rural and underserved areas—no nationwide guidance exists on best practices to develop a behavioral health workforce that can meet community need. The Behavioral Health Education of Nebraska (BHECN) can serve as an exemplar for others looking to take a multifaceted approach to develop the behavioral

The mission of the National Institute of Mental Health (NIMH) is to transform the understanding and treatment of mental illnesses through basic
and clinical research, paving the way for prevention, recovery, and cure.
This mission can only be realized if full participation in the research enterprise is open to all. Nevertheless, systemic racism and other barriers remain significant obstacles to achieving a diverse workforce. To address
these barriers, NIMH must ensure a just and equitable funding process,
support diversity-focused training opportunities, and encourage research
into mental health disparities and other areas of interest to a diverse array
of scientists.

Even before the COVID-19 pandemic, telebehavioral health (TBH) was
proving itself to be a valuable, effective tool for service delivery. The widespread adoption of its use over the past 2 years for continuity of care
should be considered one of the silver linings of the pandemic. It has the
potential to be a particularly powerful tool for providing more equitable access to care for those in rural communities if barriers to broadband access
can be addressed. In addition to providing an attractive, flexible method of
service delivery for patients and families, TBH holds appeal to the workforce as well.

The American Academy of Child and Adolescent Psychiatry (AACAP) promotes the healthy development of children, adolescents, and families
through advocacy, education, and research. This requires effectively
meeting the mental health needs of historically minoritized communities.
A diverse clinician workforce is an essential component of meeting those
needs. This article will discuss AACAP's strategic plan for diversifying the
workforce, this will be done with 3 main points: promoting diversity, equity,
and inclusion (DEI) across all mission area, creating a pipeline of child and
adolescent psychiatrists, and monitoring DEI activities and progress on an
organizational level.

CHILD AND ADOLESCENT PSYCHIATRIC CLINICS

SERIES OF RELATED INTEREST
Psychiatric Clinics
https://www.psych.theclinics.com/
Pediatric Clinics
https://www.pediatric.theclinics.com/

THE CLINICS ARE AVAILABLE ONLINE!
Access your subscription at:
www.theclinics.com

Preface

Fostering Mental Health Workforce Diversity with Courage and Creativity

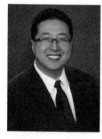 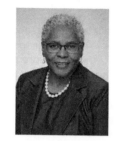

Howard Y. Liu, MD, MBA   Altha J. Stewart, MD

Editors

From 2020 to 2023, the nation experienced a series of culture shocks. In the United States, the murder of George Floyd was witnessed around the world; over 100,000 children lost a parent or caregiver during the COVID-19 pandemic; Black youth suicide rates increased at alarming rates, and LGBTQ youth faced increasing legal restrictions. Diversity initiatives offer a promising path to develop a more inclusive culture, but they must adhere to new legal guidelines to succeed. In order to anchor change, organizations must make a sustained commitment to integrated diversity and workforce development programs in child and adult mental health.

This special issue on psychiatric workforce and diversity originally sprang from the deep soil of health and social inequity in 2020. As the nation was shaken by the murder of George Floyd by law enforcement officers on May 25, 2020, this led to renewed attention to structural drivers of racism and discrimination and investment in diversity, equity, inclusion, and belonging (DEIB) offices in health care organizations. COVID-19 created a disproportionate impact on communities of color, with increased "hospitalizations, and deaths in areas where racial and ethnic minority groups live, learn, work, play and worship."[1] From 2020 to 2021, the COVID-19 pandemic caused 140,000 US youth to lose a parent or caretaker, and 65% of these losses were experienced by racial or ethnic minority families.[2] Asian American Pacific Islander communities experienced an upsurge of violence and hate crimes, exacerbated by scapegoating based on misinformation regarding the origins of the COVID-19 pandemic, with 11,500 hate incidents reported from 2020 to 2022.[3] Meanwhile, women in medicine continued to report minimal progress over a 35-year period regarding promotion to senior rank or to the role of department chair.[4] These events, layered upon centuries of historic

Child Adolesc Psychiatric Clin N Am 33 (2024) xi–xv
https://doi.org/10.1016/j.chc.2023.09.008
1056-4993/24/© 2023 Published by Elsevier Inc.

inequities, catalyzed important conversations about diversity and the psychiatric and mental health workforce.

After the original issue was published in 2022, Elsevier invited us to publish a new issue with an emphasis on the diverse needs in the child and adolescent psychiatry workforce. This is a timely opportunity for us to reflect on the rapidly changing landscape of diversity efforts in the context of societal change. We made an editorial decision to include the original articles from the 2022 issue unchanged, as the voices and ideas remain relevant, and to also include new voices that highlighted important areas of children's mental health, LGBTQ workforce, and the intersection of sports and psychiatry, which we were unable to address in the first issue.[5]

In 2023, the ecosystem of diversity initiatives is radically different than 2020. As a wellspring of DEIB initiatives arose in medical schools, and health care organizations appointed chief diversity officers, there was a backlash that changed the legal strategies for effecting change. In June 2022, the US Supreme Court ruled in *Dobbs v Jackson Women's Health Organization* that abortion was no longer a constitutionally protected right for women.[6] In June 2023, the US Supreme Court ended race-conscious admission programs at higher-education institutions across the United States, effectively ending affirmative action.[7] As of August 2023, legislators in 37 states have introduced bills to restrict gender-affirming health care for transgendered individuals, and 23 states have passed laws restricting transgender athletes' ability to participate in school sports in accordance with their gender identity.[8,9]

The cumulative impact of these legal changes has created a challenging environment for educators and organizations seeking to welcome individuals from every community. Without integration of DEIB initiatives into the culture of institutions and the daily priority of senior leaders, there is a risk of retrenchment to a status quo where the workforce does not reflect the diversity of the patients it serves. As a former President of the American Psychiatric Association and director of public mental health systems in three large urban jurisdictions, and as a former state behavioral health workforce center director in a rural state, we understand that this is not the time to make incremental change. The leaders of organized psychiatry, amateur and professional sports organizations, and health care systems have an opportunity to be ambitious and truly build and resource the structures to support a diverse mental health workforce. As we stated in our last issue, "Our collective will as leaders, educators, administrators and advocates must be sustained and amplified through many fiscal cycles, many political cycles, many leadership cycles, and many training cycles if we are to fundamentally change the workforce."[5] We stand by these words today.

In this new environment, leadership will require engagement, perseverance, creativity, courage, and humility. In order to sustain change, we must recognize that diversity policies and initiatives are national, but that they are implemented locally. Local engagement is required in every state, across political affiliations, and in urban and rural settings, as mental health leaders must listen to needs and design programs that partner with local community organizations, people with lived experience, policymakers, and mental health organizations.

Perseverance is needed to achieve long-term change in the workforce. It can take 14 years for a high school senior to become a child psychiatrist, requiring a student who is underrepresented in medicine to survive a gauntlet of obstacles from implicit bias to financial hardship to gaps in mentorship and sponsorship. During that long training period, individual program directors, chairs, and deans often turn over, requiring an institutional culture that creates, supports, and sustains DEIB policies and practices at multiple levels to avoid loss of momentum. In this issue, the article from Drs Brown, Benton, and Ng, "AACAP's Strategic Plans to Enhance the

Diversity of the Child Psychiatry and Child Mental Health Workforce Across All Mission Areas," demonstrates one example from the American Academy of Child and Adolescent Psychiatry of a professional society seeking to embed diversity principles into its structures from 1994 to the present day.

In this rapidly changing legal landscape, leaders must be creative. They must develop or adapt strategies that meet new legal standards while staying true to the vision of creating a diverse and representative mental health workforce. For example, the 2023 US Supreme Court ruling on affirmative action forbids the use of race in admission decisions at institutions of higher learning. It still allows medical schools to foster diversity in a race-neutral way, which might include recruitment of first-generation college students, outreach to students evidencing socioeconomic diversity, mentorship of students speaking multiple languages, and so forth.[10] These alternative methods have not yet been tested legally but are worth exploring. Similarly, mental health training leaders can encourage trainees to apply their expertise to careers beyond the traditional pathways of academia, private practice, and so forth. Sports psychiatry, especially the developmental and psychological impacts on youth athletes, is one such example of a burgeoning field with tremendous opportunity to showcase the diversity of needs of athletes, coaches, and staff as leaders who speak up about mental health awareness, LGBTQ inclusion, and so forth. Most of today's professional athletes began as adolescents and often describe their initial psychological challenges being overlooked or dismissed by family, coaches, and supporters as they were moving up through their chosen sport. The growing field of sport psychiatry now offers evidence-based and often preventive practices, which can be incorporated early in their athletic development to address some of the challenges that confront adolescents and might signal likelihood and risk for more serious issues later, as addressed in the article, "Sports Psychiatry: Assuring a Diverse Workforce in an Area of Increasing Professional Interest," by Stewart and colleagues.

Courage and humility will be required in equal measure in the new landscape for workforce diversity in the years ahead. The authors do not doubt that there will be ongoing legal battles at the state and federal level to define which strategies are permitted for increasing diversity in workforce development programs at institutions of higher learning. This will require mental health leaders to stay current on policies and to try emerging strategies in this rapidly shifting legal and regulatory environment. It will require leaders in mental health advocacy to work in a bipartisan fashion and build the diverse coalitions that can underscore the importance of achieving a diverse mental health workforce in every community. For example, as LGBTQ youth are increasingly facing restrictions in many states, we must prioritize training more LGBTQ child psychiatrists who can support them through this difficult landscape, as described by Ramos and colleagues in "Recruitment, Retention, and Wellbeing of LGBTQ Child Psychiatrists and Child Mental Health Workforce." And it will require the humility to acknowledge that mental health professionals must make their own decisions about whether to stay in communities where they or their loved ones feel less welcomed or where their mental health practices face legal jeopardy.

Some efforts will fail, while others succeed, and we must learn from both. This is a time when leaders must be nimble. Despite the challenges, we are optimistic as we see leaders working across generations to protect, resource, and embed the principles of diversity into institutional DNA. As attorney, author, and former First Lady of the United States, Michelle Obama, states, "Find people who will make you better." It is the privilege and the responsibility of leaders to empower, sponsor, and engage future generations of diverse mental health professionals. We must help every community feel welcome in health care, and we hope that this issue will take us a little farther along the path to achieving that goal.

CONFLICT OF INTEREST/DISCLOSURE

Dr Stewart is a consultant/speaker for Otsuka Pharmaceuticals; Dr Liu is a consultant/speaker for Medscape.

ACKNOWLEDGMENTS

The authors acknowledge Arghavan Salles, MD, PhD, Special Advisor for DEI Programs at Stanford University Department of Medicine and Senior Research Scholar, Clayman Institute for Gender Research; Clinical Associate Professor, Medicine–Gastroenterology and Hepatology, Stanford Medicine; Sheritta A. Strong, MD, MBA, Assistant Vice Chancellor for Inclusion, UNMC; Director of Diversity, Equity, and Inclusion, UNMC Department of Psychiatry; Associate Professor, UNMC COM; Ruth S. Shim, MD, MPH, Associate Dean for Diverse and Inclusive Education, UC Davis School of Medicine; Luke & Grace Kim Professor in Cultural Psychiatry; Director of Cultural Psychiatry and Professor in the Department of Psychiatry and Behavioral Sciences, Sacramento, California; Terri C. Jackson, JD, Executive Director, Women's National Basketball Players Association, New York, New York.

Howard Y. Liu, MD, MBA
Department of Psychiatry
University of Nebraska Medical Center
985575 Nebraska Medical Center
Omaha, NE 68198-5575, USA

Altha J. Stewart, MD
Division of Public and Community Psychiatry
Center for Youth Advocacy and Well-Being
Women's National Basketball Association
University of Tennessee Health Science Center
66 North Pauline Street, Suite 205
Memphis, TN 38163, USA

E-mail addresses:
hyliu@unmc.edu (H.Y. Liu)
astewa59@uthsc.edu (A.J. Stewart)

REFERENCES

1. Centers for Disease Control and Prevention. January 25, 2022. Health equity considerations and racial and ethnic minority groups. Available at: https://www.cdc.gov/coronavirus/2019-ncov/community/health-equity/race-ethnicity.html#:~:text=Impact%20of%20Racial%20Inequities%20on%20Our%20Nation's%20Health,-Racism%2C%20either%20structural&text=COVID%2D19%20data%20shows%20that,with%20non%2DHispanic%20White%20populations. Accessed March 6, 2022.
2. NIDA. The Hidden U.S. COVID-19 Pandemic: Orphaned Children—More than 140,000 U.S. children lost a primary or secondary caregiver due to the COVID-19 pandemic. National Institute on Drug Abuse website. October 7, 2021. Available at: https://nida.nih.gov/news-events/news-releases/2021/10/the-hidden-us-covid-19-pandemic-orphaned-children-more-than-140000-us-children-lost-a-primary-

or-secondary-caregiver-due-to-the-covid-19-pandemic. Accessed September 20, 2023.

3. Yellow Horse AJ, Chen T. Two years and thousands of voices: what community-generated data tells us about anti-AAPI hate. Stop AAPI Hate. 2022. Available at: https://stopaapihate.org/wp-content/uploads/2023/06/22-SAH-NationalReport-July-F.pdf. Accessed September 20, 2023.

4. Richter KP, Clark L, Wick JA, et al. Women physicians and promotion in academic medicine. N Engl J Med 2020;383(22):2148–57.

5. Liu HY, Stewart AJ. The diversity of the mental health workforce requires a sustained commitment. Psychiatr Clin North Am 2022;45(2). xiii–xvii.

6. Romo V. A year after Dobbs and the end of Roe v. Wade, there's chaos and confusion. National Public Radio. June 24, 2023. Available at: https://www.npr.org/2023/06/24/1183639093/abortion-ban-dobbs-roe-v-wade-anniversary-confusion. Accessed September 19, 2023.

7. Totenberg N. Supreme Court guts affirmative action, effectively ending race-conscious admissions. National Public Radio. June 29, 2023. Available at: https://www.npr.org/2023/06/29/1181138066/affirmative-action-supreme-court-decision. Accessed September 19, 2023.

8. Wolfe J, Goldenberg S, Flynn D. The rise of anti-trans bills in the US. Reuters, 2023. Available at: https://www.reuters.com/graphics/USA-HEALTHCARE/TRANS-BILLS/zgvorreyapd/. Accessed September 19, 2023.

9. Barnes K. Transgender athlete laws by state: legislation, science, more. ESPN.com, 2023. Available at: https://www.espn.com/espn/story/_/id/38209262/transgender-athlete-laws-state-legislation-science. Accessed September 20, 2023.

10. Adashi EY, Gruppuso PA, Cohen IG. Affirmative action ruled unconstitutional: options for building a diverse health care workforce. JAMA 2023;330(11):1031–2.

Profiles in Wisdom
A Survey of Leading Psychiatrists to Inform the Diversity of the Future Psychiatric Workforce

Michael O. Mensah, MD, MPH[a],*, Amira Collison, MD[b],
Dennis Dacarett-Galeano, MD, MPH[b], Altha J. Stewart, MD[c],1

KEYWORDS

- Mental health • Diversity • Equity • Inclusion • Workforce • Organized psychiatry

KEY POINTS

- Long-standing challenges facing our nation's mental health system require more effective strategies to furnish a workforce whose diversity matches the increasingly diverse population we serve.
- Current and former system leaders can offer expert guidance informed by their experiences and perspectives when given the opportunity. Their professional journeys to leadership in this area provide helpful context and unique insight into addressing and resolving issues of justice, including workforce diversity, equity, and inclusion in psychiatry.
- These experts agree that significant policy changes are needed to improve psychiatric workforce diversity. Implementing change will require that disparate groups—including regulatory, accrediting, and funding bodies as well as academic institutions—work together to achieve this goal.
- Financial considerations must always be included in policy and advocacy efforts intended to significantly change the structure of mental health care systems related to reducing disparities and achieving equity.

The syndemic of social injustice, structural racism, and COVID-19 exposed and exacerbated long-standing mental health inequities in the United States, prompting stewards of mental health care to undergo a vocational, often painful, self-examination.[1–3]

This article originally appeared in *Psychiatric Clinics*, Volume 45 Issue 2, June 2022.
[a] National Clinician Scholars Program, Department of Medicine, Yale University School of Medicine, New Haven, CT, USA; [b] Department of Psychiatry and Biobehavioral Sciences, Semel Institute for Neuroscience and Human Behavior, University of California, Los Angeles, CA, USA; [c] Division of Public and Community Psychiatry and Office of Community Health Engagement, College of Medicine, University of Tennessee Health Science Center, Memphis, TN, USA
[1] Present address: 66 North Pauline St., Suite 205 Memphis, TN 38163, USA
* Corresponding author. National Clinician Scholars Program, Yale University School of Medicine, 333 Cedar Street, SHM IE-66, New Haven, CT 06510.
E-mail address: mim159@mail.harvard.edu

Child Adolesc Psychiatric Clin N Am 33 (2024) 1–15
https://doi.org/10.1016/j.chc.2023.06.002
1056-4993/24/© 2023 Elsevier Inc. All rights reserved.

This moment has felt especially urgent for trainees, early career providers, and professionals as well as some in organizational leadership to escalate advocacy for vulnerable populations.[4,5] The anxious zeitgeist energizes efforts to create roadmaps to mental health equity. But the tremendous challenge of effectively confronting inequity will require longer-term commitments not yet made—or even recognized—by most leadership in mental health. Without such a commitment, sustainable equity will remain out of reach.

Short of securing long-term commitment, how can trainees, early career providers, and their stewards increase the odds of future equity? One answer is to increase psychiatric workforce diversity and orienting institutions toward the change that diverse workforce demands. Diverse workforces in medicine increase the number of providers available to underresourced populations.[6,7] This is especially important in psychiatry, where providers are less likely to take insurance and who care for less wealthy patients.[8,9]

Diversity alone, however, will not orient institutions toward equity. Organizations must center diversity through structural inclusion, thereby empowering implementation of equitable reform. A corollary is that effective reform cannot be limited to budget-positive or budget-neutral initiatives—equity requires investment. These are not yet common practices, so diverse advocate-providers who seek antiracist reform must have savvy in order to navigate structures and win support. Acquiring savvy without corresponding experience requires wisdom and historical accounts from experienced, successful advocates, and leaders in mental health.

A search conducted indicated little evidence in the current literature of a historical account responsive to the current need for organizational memory and know-how to meet the opportunity for improved diversity, inclusion and, eventually, equity. Of note, one article addressed a different but related question regarding diversity leadership within academic departments.[4] In response to this gap in the literature, the authors interviewed psychiatrists with extensive organizational experience to contextualize and inform next steps in creating and empowering a more diverse workforce in psychiatry.

SURVEY DESIGN

We interviewed eight expert attending psychiatrists who have championed diversity, equity, and inclusion in their careers. Their diverse perspectives (racial identity, gender, sexual orientation, and practice settings) inform their recommendations for the future psychiatric workforce. All interviews were conducted over Zoom, and we note when data gathering took place over multiple sessions. The interviewees included a coauthor on this manuscript (A.J.S.). In the interview summary, we provide a context for each expert's recommendations and "lessons learned." We then synthesized several common themes from all interviews in our discussion. These talking points were the general guidelines for each interview:

- How would you describe past diversity efforts in psychiatry, how those efforts have changed, and where you see psychiatry heading in the future?
- What do you think are the most significant barriers in achieving diversity in the psychiatric workforce?
- What do you believe are promising next steps or interventions that we can take now to further diversity the field of psychiatry?

The following results synthesize several hours of interviews with each expert. We thank each interviewee for their time and candor.

RESULTS: INTERVIEWS 1 TO 8
Interview 1

Subject: Francis Lu, MD, DLFAPA, Luke and Grace Kim Professor in Cultural Psychiatry, Emeritus, Professor of Clinical Psychiatry, Emeritus, University of California, Davis. associate chair for medical student education at UC Davis Health

Interviewers: Michael O. Mensah, MD, MPH; Amira Collison, MD; Dennis Dacarett-Galeano, MD, MPH; and Altha J. Stewart, MD

Location and date: Zoom, 9/26/21

Francis Lu, MD, DLFAPA, is considered the father of cultural psychiatry. After training at Mount Sinai, he was recruited to the Department of Psychiatry at the San Francisco General Hospital, in part because of leadership's interest in Japanese culture. After becoming unit chief, Lu started his Asia Pacific–focused inpatient program and eventually developed Latino-; human immunodeficiency virus/AIDS-; woman-; lesbian, gay, bisexual, and transgender (LGBT)-; and African American–focused inpatient programs at San Francisco General Hospital.[10,11] Withstanding pressure from leadership at the Department of Public Health to close the wards, his service won the Certificate of Significant Achievement from the American Psychiatric Association (APA), the Creativity in Psychiatric Education Award from the American College of Psychiatrists, and an Excellence in Cultural Competence Award from the San Francisco Department of Public Health. It is no exaggeration that the field of cultural psychiatry grew out of his groundbreaking clinical work.

Dr Lu's influence extends to medical training internationally. From 2009 to 2012, he served as a founding member of the steering group for the Association of American Medical Colleges Group on Diversity and Inclusion. He has worked tirelessly to guide programs adapting to new Accreditation Council for Graduate Medical Education requirements—to "recruit and retain a diverse and inclusive workforce" and other similar requirements.[12] Dr Lu played a key part in establishing these requirements, with which programs must comply or risk sanction or probation. As such, many have sought out Dr Lu's wisdom and mentorship. He continues to lead efforts to assure that required changes are made in accordance with the new guidelines.

Accordingly, the first lesson Dr Lu imparts on current and future advocates is to be detail-oriented regarding policy. The decision to implement policy can hinge on seemingly small details. For example, he notes that changes to promotion guidelines to value diversity-related activities increased their value to untenured faculty, thereby increasing the department's overall contribution to diversity efforts. Reminding medical school deans and department chairs of diversity's centrality to the educational mission ensured that such policy "had teeth." To that end, Dr Lu also recommends empowering policy changes by involving institutional leaders in ongoing diversity efforts, especially within training programs. Leadership usually has wide discretion as to how diversity initiatives are supported, funded, and implemented. Their involvement can accelerate progress through top-down endorsement and empowerment. Finally, Dr Lu recommends that future leaders stay involved in organizations—despite their shortcomings and sometimes anachronistic beliefs—because they wield tremendous resources that, directed correctly, will result in achieving equity in our systems and institutions.

Interview 2

Subject: Rahn Kennedy Bailey, 113th president of the National Medical Association (2012–13), former APA minority and underrepresented trustee (2019–2021), current department chair and assistant dean for community engagement at LSU School of Medicine

Interviewers: Michael O. Mensah, MD, MPH, and Amira Collison, MD

Location and date: Zoom, 10/8/21

Dr Rahn Bailey has been an advocate for racial justice within psychiatry since becoming a medical student at University of Texas, where he served as Student National Medical Association chapter president and the only African American on its admissions committee. His career has taken him across the country, from Texas and New Haven to North Carolina, California, and now Louisiana. Throughout, structural forces have decreased access to and quality of health care for African American patients. Much like the marginalization of psychiatry within the house of medicine, African Americans with mental illness face similar delegitimization of their illnesses within the mental health system.[13–15]

Dr Bailey researched treatment of schizophrenia during the 1990s and early 2000s, when atypical antipsychotics emerged as a popular alternative to typical antipsychotics due to their more favorable side-effect profile. Their expense and scarcity, however, forced providers treating Black and brown patients in publicly funded systems to advocate extensively to achieve psychiatric "pharmacoequity"—or access to the best medications for mental illness regardless of their race and ethnicity or socioeconomic status.[16] Dr Bailey describes this fight as "ferocious" and with stakes as high as the drug's cost: second-generation antipsychotics made up one-fourth of the Medicaid drug budget as recently as the late 2000s.[17] Notably, Dr Bailey recounted comparing antipsychotic access to antibiotic access to highlight the disparity, an example of scaffolding a stigmatized concept to one less stigmatized to vividly illustrate inequity.

Dr Bailey offered four points for the next generation of clinician-advocates to consider: financial implications, shifting emphasis from only diversity to diversity, equity and inclusion, outreach strategies to expose minority students to medicine and psychiatry earlier in their education, and winning nonminority ally support for diversity, equity, and inclusion efforts. Financial considerations are increasingly important, because many workplace diversity, equity, and inclusion initiatives will require an initial investment from leadership and compensation for the labor required to achieve workforce diversity. Such investment paves the road from diversity to diversity, equity, and inclusion, alongside evidence-based policies and practices that help individuals not just survive but also advance to inclusive leadership in psychiatry. Without inclusion, underrepresented minorities often feel "tokenized," rendering any sense of failure as confirmation of negative stereotypes associated with their identity. This stereotype threat raises stakes and anxiety unnecessarily, thereby decreasing working memory.[18] Finally, champions of diversity, equity, and inclusion must include nonminority allies in their efforts in order to build strong and effective coalitions. Sharing the aforementioned labor of system change reduces the minority tax, because having underrepresented minorities do the enormous and necessary amount of diversity work before implementing inclusion that values their work penalizes them for their labor and puts them at risk for burnout and leaving the organization.[19,20]

Finally, Dr Bailey recounts his own personal journey to psychiatry, which has come full circle. Having started as a college student involved in a community pipeline program, he now leads a local community mentorship program. As such, he urges upcoming psychiatrists to become involved in their community to prepare, inspire, and attract students from historically marginalized communities into the field of psychiatry.

Interview 3

Subject: Jack Drescher, MD, Clinical Professor of Psychiatry, Columbia University, College of Physicians and Surgeons, Faculty Member, Columbia University Center for Psychoanalytic Training and Research, Clinical Supervisor and Adjunct Professor, New York University Postdoctoral Program in Psychotherapy and Psychoanalysis, and Training and Supervising Analyst at William Alanson White Institute
    Interviewers: Michael O. Mensah, MD, MPH, and Dennis Dacarett-Galeano, MD, MPH
    Location and date: Zoom, 10/15/2021

    Dr Jack Drescher pursued his training as a psychiatrist at a pivotal moment in LGBT and queer/questioning (LGBTQ) history. He recalls being pathologized for his sexuality during a 1979 interview for an internship by a psychoanalyst at a prestigious New York City academic medical center. Although he knew that homosexuality was no longer considered a disorder in the *Diagnostic and Statistical Manual of Mental Disorders* (*DSM*) as of 1973, he did not know many psychoanalysts considered its omission controversial. He went on to train at St. Vincent's in New York City for his internship and King's County Hospital for residency, where glaring social differences between the community and the providers treating them piqued his interest in inequity.

    At a turning point in the AIDS crisis, these personal experiences and observations compelled him to advocacy. Dr Drescher began serving on the Gay, Lesbian, and Bisexual committee and the AIDS committee of the local district branch of the APA and went on to serve as president of the APA New York County Psychiatric Society. Through the APA, he has written numerous position statements and served as a media spokesperson on LGBTQ issues. Most recently, he has served on the APA *DSM* (Fifth Edition) Sexual and Gender Identity Disorders Workgroup and serves on the World Health Organization Working Group on the Classification of Sexual Disorders and Sexual Health, addressing sex and gender diagnoses in the World Health Organization forthcoming (2018) revisions of the *International Classification of Diseases, Eleventh Revision*. He is emeritus editor of the *Journal of Gay & Lesbian Mental Health* and serves on editorial boards of seven academic journals. In discussing efforts in activism, he acknowledges that there is grief and encourages others to intentionally seek out community in their advocacy efforts.

    Citing his own example of his experiences within the psychoanalytic tradition, Dr Drescher states that some of the barriers toward achieving equity, diversity, and inclusion in psychiatry are due to the lack of a reconciliation process regarding a legacy of historical injustice in psychiatry. Reconciliation requires recognition, so Dr Drescher urges all psychiatrists to willfully recognize current and historical injustices, even if it makes them uncomfortable. He further asserts that the field will not get a consensus on issues regarding diversity, equity, and inclusion if there is a lack of representation from all the diverse communities. He urges members of minority and marginalized groups to look beyond their identities for allies. His continued work and commitment to the issue serves as a model for the next generation of psychiatrist-advocates who identify as LGBTQ and will support expansion of the field's ability to assure diversity efforts include representation from this community as well.

Interview 4

Subject: Nada Stotland, MD, 135th president of the American Psychiatric Association (2008–2009), professor of psychiatry and of obstetrics and gynecology at Rush Medical College
    Interviewers: Michael O. Mensah, MD, MPH, and Amira Collison, MD
    Location and date: Zoom, 10/17/2021

Nada Stotland, MD, has witnessed several forms of inequity since her APA career began in the 1970s. After the *Roe v Wade* decision, Dr Stotland joined the Illinois Psychiatric Society and started its Women's Mental Health Group, where her focus was—and continues to be—women's issues, including abortion rights. Stotland's advocacy accelerated her advancement, and she was eventually appointed to the APA Committee on Women.

One notable incident concerned data indicating that some psychiatrists had inappropriate relationships with patients. Leadership feared the data threatened psychiatry's image. With a perspective inclusive of such misconduct's victims, Dr Stotland successfully reframed the survey as an opportunity to lead all of medicine, eventually advocating for organizational examination of the issue. Her advocacy eventually led to the APA Assembly, in 1993, explicitly prohibiting sexual contact between a psychiatrist and former patient, with no statute of limitations specified.[21] The APA president was so impressed with her, he invited her to the national board meetings. There, she witnessed male domination of board meetings, to the point that she felt she could not speak at the meeting unless spoken to first.

During this time, Dr Stotland also witnessed what she describes as "the clumsy beginnings of the APA's racial discussions." For example, a chair of the Committee of Black Psychiatrists became an observer-consultant—also a guest of the board—and nonvoting member of the board following the 1969 walk-in by Black psychiatrist members. He usually said nothing and was rarely asked his opinion. On one occasion however, the Black consultant—as the only Black person at the table—brought up an instance of racism within the APA. In response, the sitting APA president said, "I've never seen a racist thing happen at this organization!" The president was incredibly dismissive, offended at the accusation that there was racism in the APA. The conflict escalated, demonstrating to Dr Stotland not only the risk informing the decision of Black members of the APA to not speak up or express their concerns about racial issues but also the negative consequences of not including marginalized people in these important discussions.

Her recommendations for the future include encouraging young equity advocates to focus on persuasion, the emotional component of changing minds that changes cultures. Her experience garnering support for clinical guidelines around abortion informed this advice.[22,23] She learned from a colleague to shift from accusing the audience of not caring about women's issues to making the audience feel good for embracing knowledge they already had to achieve the best outcome. This allowed individuals to harness existing self-concepts and move them toward systemic change and more equitable practices.

Second, Dr Stotland wants younger psychiatrists to acknowledge the different perspectives held by their older peers regarding racism and other issues of social justice in health care. She readily admits that she continues to learn about racism in psychiatry, despite her vast experience working with minority groups within the APA. As such, she imagines activities that bring racially discriminatory experiences to life for White folks. Similar to drug company exhibits that simulate auditory hallucinations for those without psychosis, she imagines that simulating racially based experiences for empathic White people will change their perspective and that they will advocate for those people in positions of power in the APA to support minority members attaining positions of power and welcome their ideas and concerns.

Interview 5

Subject: David C. Henderson, MD, psychiatrist-in-chief at Boston Medical Center (BMC) and professor and chair of psychiatry at Boston University School of Medicine (BUSM)

Interviewers: Michael O. Mensah, MD, MPH, and Amira Collison, MD
Location and date: Zoom, 10/20/2021

Dr David C. Henderson is a leading figure in academic psychiatry, currently leading the Department of Psychiatry at BMC. Despite Henderson's numerous career accomplishments—including codirecting the National Institute of Mental Health Institutional Research Training Grants (T32) BUSM/Global Psychiatry Clinical Research Fellowship and previously directing the Chester M. Pierce Division of Global Psychiatry, the MGH Schizophrenia Clinical and Research Program, and the Harvard Program in Refugee Trauma at MGH—he notes several challenges. Henderson was so struck by the "appalling" lack of diversity in the BMC Department of Psychiatry during his first chief's meeting that he walked out, returning minutes later to emphasize that if he was to lead BMC psychiatry, the department, including its leadership, should reflect Boston's diversity. Six years after that demand, his department's diversity has dramatically increased, thanks to his intentional recruitment and selection of diverse faculty and trainees and advocating for their promotion and retention in departmental leadership roles. Henderson notes that the visibility of the department's diversity serves to attract more diverse trainees and faculty, creating an environment where people of all backgrounds feel included, rather than tokenized.

Henderson believes diversity should be prioritized because of the disparities in the quality and access to mental health care services in marginalized populations.[24] As documented in "Mental Health: A Report of the Surgeon General" and its supplement, "Mental Health, Culture, Race and Ethnicity," racial and ethnic minorities have less access to mental health services than do Whites, are less likely to receive needed care, and are more likely to receive poor quality care when treated.[25,26] Therefore, Henderson urges that we need more diverse psychiatric providers to allow patients the opportunity to work with a provider who looks like them and may bring a shared background or life experience to the treatment that will improve the quality of care they receive as part of a historically underserved group.

An internationally renowned expert in schizophrenia and antipsychotic therapy, Henderson has found that Black patients are more likely to be prescribed older generations of antipsychotics or antipsychotics with poorer side-effect profiles, such as weight gain and hyperlipidemia, despite population-based data that suggest that providers need to be mindful of these metabolic side effects when prescribing atypical antipsychotics.[27] Similarly, Henderson has demonstrated evidence of patients' varying susceptibilities to metabolic side effects based on race,[28] including evidence that clozapine may have more metabolic side effects for African Americans and Hispanics than Whites.[29]

Considering the increasing awareness of the health care disparities affecting his institution's surrounding communities, Henderson provided an example of an impactful initiative his hospital system implemented. The health equity accelerator collects population data and then finds and addresses areas of health disparity in communities.[30] Henderson notes this initiative spans all hospital system departments and specialties and believes such a system should be in place across the country.

Additionally, Henderson believes, "we need to expose more young people to Black psychiatrists," because, as a child, he was exposed to Black psychiatrists through his mother, who worked in a nearby hospital as a nurse. He encourages more minority psychiatrists to interact with, guide, and mentor the future generation of minority physicians through pipeline programs that guide underrepresented minority students into fields of medicine.

Interview 6

Subject: Robert Rohrbaugh, MD, professor of psychiatry, associate dean for global health education, deputy dean for professionalism and leadership, and deputy chair for education and career development, Department of Psychiatry, Yale School of Medicine

Interviewers: Michael O. Mensah, MD, MPH, and Dennis Dacarett-Galeano, MD, MPH

Location and date: Zoom, 10/21/2021

A graduate of Franklin and Marshall College, Yale School of Medicine, and the Yale psychiatry residency and geriatric psychiatry fellowship programs, Dr Rohrbaugh joined the Yale Department of Psychiatry faculty in 1988. Coming from a disadvantaged community in Pennsylvania Dutch Country, he was elated by the opportunities Yale provided. He started his journey into advocacy after realizing 10 years into his career at Yale that many of his colleagues of color did not experience the institution in the positive way he had, prompting him to listen more attentively. He has since prioritized diversity due to the systemic health inequities we see in our health care system and accordingly has committed much of his career as Yale program director and deputy chair for education to training a generation of psychiatrists who can change the field by dismantling institutional racism and White supremacy–based treatment systems.[31]

Most recently, Dr Rohrbaugh has worked to educate Yale medical students and residents in global health and has worked with colleagues at Xiangya School of Medicine in Changsha, Hunan Province, People's Republic of China, to develop a competency-based model for postgraduate (residency) education. This model has heavily influenced the Chinese national model for residency training. He was named the founding director of the Yale School of Medicine Office of International Medical Student Education in 2008. Again, taking a wide perspective led to a career change: in 2015, having noted the irony that global health education is largely discussed by educators in high-income countries, Dr Rohrbaugh cofounded the Bellagio Global Health Education Initiative, with an explicit goal of bringing global health education leaders from high-, middle-, and low-income countries together to developed global health curricula that could be implemented worldwide. He cites many influential peers and leaders that have guided his understanding and advocacy: Drs Flavia D'Souza, Myra Mathis, Jessica Isom, Helena Hansen, Ayana Jordan, Enrico Castillo, and John Krystal, among others. Of note, many of these leaders are junior to Dr Rohrbaugh, demonstrating his structural humility despite hierarchical differences in power.[31]

Despite this advocacy, he reflects on the data that demonstrate little movement since the 1970s regarding inclusion of underrepresented minorities. He recommends that the field more often center marginalized voices, that leaders leverage their power when they can, and that people discuss issues around equity, diversity, and inclusion through the lens of their value system. Additionally, he notes that leaders use the information gleaned from listening to marginalized voices to inform clinical, training, and research practices moving forward.

Interview 7

Subject: Kenneth Thompson, MD, medical director and founder of the Pennsylvania Psychiatric Leadership Council (PPLC); past president, American Association for Social Psychiatry, at-large representative, board of the American Association for Community Psychiatrists

Interviewer: Michael O. Mensah, MD, MPH
Location and date: Zoom, 10/27/2021

Dr Thompson's advocacy journey started like many health outcomes—before his birth. His father, a physician himself, was raised in Boston by a man who became wealthy through cotton trading in the Jim Crow South. He joined the Medical Committee for Human Rights soon after the junior Dr Thompson was born, traveling down to the Deep South as an advocate for civil rights, despite the recent Freedom Summer murders, where James Chaney, a Black man, as well as Andrew Goodman and Michael Henry Schwerner, two White men, went missing and were later found slain by the Ku Klux Klan.

Risking life for justice—and having his mother support the effort despite the risk—impressed on Dr Thompson a sense of duty and an obligation to "meet patients where they are at." While attending BUSM, Dr Thompson was struck by the "excessive death zones" surrounding Boston's hospitals.[32] At first, he believed these geographic disparities were somehow explained by health care access, despite the proximity of the hospitals. His assumptions were challenged, however, during his time in Scotland—his matrilineal country of origin—where he learned about *The Black Report*, which demonstrated a dose-dependent relationship that associated social factors like socioeconomic class and control over one's vocational environment with several health outcomes.[33]

Since this observation, Dr Thompson has emphasized to colleagues the enormous impact social factors—including structural racism—can have on health. The PPLC created fellowships for public psychiatry intended to work with residency directors to make Pennsylvania more attractive to racial minority trainees and aim to build the "best system of public mental health care" in the country. Since its inception 15 years ago, PPLC has survived thanks to the advocacy efforts of Estelle Richman, former Pennsylvania secretary of the Department of Welfare and chief operating officer of the US Department of Housing and Urban Development, and more junior leaders like Dr Leon Cushenberry, a Black psychiatrist and National Clinician Scholar active with PPLC.

Building coalitions in a context not always friendly to antiracist solutions has taught Dr Thompson several lessons. First, he notes from his positionality as a White, cis-identifying, heterosexual man that other people who look like him—and thus are structurally positioned to wield power—will be less threatened when delivering antiracist messaging than a Black, trans-identifying, gay woman. As such, he suggests a model of antiracist advocacy where folks in the majority—especially White men—have at least as much as and possibly more "skin in the game" than Black folks.

What does this commitment look like? Dr Thompson recommends that the next generation pay close attention to how systems are financed, including wages across the spectrum from physicians to others in the workforce.[34,35] At the highest levels, individual wealth derives from pain and suffering, and, when this pain and suffering results from preventable social ills, we have a duty as altruistic healers to prevent them. As such, we should advocate for clinical as well as social conditions for healing. Throughout his career, he has seen the profit motive supersede the overall healing motive,[36] leading to the injustices he tries to address through social initiatives.

Interview 8

Subject: Altha J. Stewart, MD, 145th and first African American president of APA (2018–2019), associate professor of psychiatry; and director, public and community psychiatry; and director of the Center for Health in Justice Involved Youth, at the University of Tennessee Health Science Center in Memphis

Interviewers: Michael O. Mensah, MD, MPH; Amira Collison, MD; and Dennis Dacarett-Galeano, MD, MPH

Location and date: Zoom, 10/26/2021 and 11/11/2021

The first African American president in the APA's 177-year history, Altha J. Stewart, MD, combines charisma, intelligence, and triple consciousness as a Black woman to leave her indelible footprint on the field of psychiatry. Stewart credits her family and upbringing for instilling in her a natural desire for public service. Through delivery of mental health care in the private and public sectors of Philadelphia, New York City, Detroit, and Memphis, Stewart has touched the lives of countless individuals with mental illness and their families across the country. Working with historically marginalized and underserved minority communities is Dr Stewart's "calling." Throughout her career, she has worked tirelessly to secure "a seat at the table" to amplify the voices of minority communities. Reflecting on her experiences adjacent to power, Stewart recalls an "anything but race" mentality, notably from administrators and board members who chose to avoid race discussions due to their own discomfort. It is this aversive racism, however, that enables health inequities, oppression, and structural violence to persist at the core of our health institutions.[37] Stewart refused to let these discussions die, utilizing her leadership roles to force acknowledgment of the inequities that run rampant in minority communities, helping groups, including APA, to move closer toward becoming antiracist organizations.

The syndemic of social injustice, health inequities highlighting structural racism, and COVID-19 meant that groups like APA could no longer avoid a leading role in addressing workforce issues related to diversity, equity and inclusion. Stewart recalled a similar moment in May 1969, when Black psychiatrists, led by Dr Chester M. Pierce, demanded a meeting with the APA Board of Trustees, presenting a list of 10 demands to the organization, including demanding the APA acknowledge racism as a mental health problem, deny membership to psychiatrists who practiced racial discrimination, and work to desegregate all public and private mental health facilities in the United States.[38] In fact, Dr Alvin Poussaint, a dean at Harvard Medical School, who once advocated for APA to recognize extreme prejudice as a mental illness, was berated for suggesting that racism be considered a psychotic delusional disorder.[39]

One barrier Stewart notes in achieving diversity, equity, and inclusion in psychiatry is its long-standing history of silence toward racial injustice. In her presidential address, Stewart called out the APA for remaining silent during the *Brown v Board of Education* Supreme Court decision, despite the urging of prominent APA members like Dr Charles Prudhomme, the first Black elected to office in the APA. She stated, "[b]y declining to engage in this 'social' issue, the APA missed an opportunity to make a statement about the negative psychological effects of racism. proven to be more than a 'social' issue."[40] Stewart urges the next generation of psychiatrists to continue speaking out on how racism and social determinants affect the psychological health of our patients and to make effective change to assure diversity, inclusion, and equity in the future psychiatric workforce.

MAIN THEMES FROM INTERVIEWS
Psychiatrists Must Engage with Communities in Order To Effectively Serve Marginalized Groups

Each interviewee demonstrated awareness of how their constellation of identities—race, gender, sexual orientation, profession, age, education, and other dimensions—informed their career journey. This self-awareness enabled earnest engagement with their communities and those opposing the change they wanted to make.

Acknowledgment of differences between professionals and frontline workers demonstrates situational awareness and informs credibility, which facilitates collaboration for system change. Indeed, self-awareness of social positionality signals empathy and insight regarding specific barriers marginalized groups experience.

Successful Advocacy Requires a Detail-Oriented Approach

Organizations often use detailed, expert-informed policy to guide their action. In order to redirect an organization, advocates must take advantage of opportunities to change policy by knowing target policy as well as its authors. This often requires deep engagement, a difficult task for those dissatisfied with the organization's direction. Well-informed policy advocates, however, can use their detail-informed expertise to reshape policy by showing how proposed changes might align policy more closely with the mission of the organization.

Know and Respect History, Especially Living History

We should ensure we learn the history of racism within our profession, if only to better understand those practices, which supported racism's survival within psychiatry. Most of this history is not recorded—another well-known tactic of racism—so we should engage more seasoned members of our profession, who often know the history and possess the wisdom that not only prevents history from repeating itself but also informs a more diverse future. We then must use this wisdom to contextualize acknowledgment of systemic racism within our health care systems and to inform the ways in which we deliver care in order to make effective change.

Use a Multimodal Approach to Problem-solving, Then Collaborate

Both Dr Henderson and Dr Bailey encountered inequity regarding atypical antipsychotic access for their patients. Dr Bailey advocated through organized psychiatry and industry, whereas Dr Henderson used research to illustrate the inequity. These strategies synergized, potentiating the effort: research challenging claims of cost ineffectiveness in Medicaid populations was followed by increased access to atypical antipsychotics.

Use Persuasion to Achieve Change

Drs Stotland and Stewart, both APA presidents, emphasized the difficulty in moving systems toward equity. There are several barriers to this goal: the zero-sum mindset of racism,[41] confusion between equality and equity,[42] and being associated with "woke-ism" and other distortions of health equity efforts. Both presidents cautioned against sacrificing persuasiveness for the sake of impressing the soundness of an argument on an audience whose opinion is at stake. Although argumentation matters—as discussed previously—its delivery and other rhetorical elements can mitigate or augment the risk of an audience feeling bad about who they are during attempts to win support. This is especially true when discussing issues surrounding racial, gender, and other forms of equity. No matter how just or sound the argument, if the audience's defensiveness prevents them from hearing the argument, it will not change their mind. If that is not the goal of the communication, so be it. But if changing minds is the goal, the challenge of persuasion is to have your target audience associate "feeling good" with your ask. Positive reinforcement is highly persuasive.

Follow the Money

In almost every interview, financial considerations were mentioned. Regardless of size, organizational change will require financing. This need must be explicitly acknowledged for any policy to be considered antiracist. Additionally, medical education rarely includes financial or structural literacy as a competency, so any aspiring leader must seek this knowledge—from both mentors and written materials—to become skilled in understanding its role in system change.

Recommendations

1. Create more opportunities for these conversations between more seasoned psychiatrists and their young colleagues. It can be formal mentoring or an open exchange of ideas and solutions to some of the challenges facing the field going forward and allow for the passing of wisdom to the next generation. Encouraging more discussion among multigenerational teams and working together to create new and shared experiences involving planning for the future of the field will bring the best ideas for creating the workforce we need.
2. Identify leaders and senior faculty in academic psychiatry programs to work with junior faculty. Move beyond pipelines and create pathways that ensure diverse faculty members have access to opportunities to succeed in the career paths they choose. These opportunities for exchange of ideas must be value added, in terms of relationship to promotion, tenure, and other higher-level options, for faculty members of diverse backgrounds with interest in working with diverse populations and communities.
3. Seek to learn the historical injustices that brought us to the disparities and inequities we are dealing with today and build systems of training, clinical care, and research that will eliminate such injustice.
4. Make resources available for doing this work. Most of the interviewees recounted making most of the changes with minimal support. If this work is valuable, it must be funded.

SUMMARY

For the past 2 years, we have witnessed the COVID-19 pandemic reveal and synergize with long-standing racial inequities to create a syndemic, which has drawn attention to those inequities. To inform future action, eight experts offered their wisdom about how psychiatry might take advantage of the moment. Some of those pearls of wisdom are summarized. They all emphasized that future psychiatrists must be engaged with these communities to properly care for them. Each interviewer was a trailblazer and change agent in their area of expertise, committed to facing challenges instead of avoiding or minimizing them—no matter the consequences.

Such courage under fire, unfortunately, was not a common trait among many of their peers, which is why the opportunity to speak with them and ask sensitive questions in frank ways inspired the authors on this writing team. Indeed, the authors agree that it will help move the work forward if those with experience and power are not afraid to talk about racism but instead face the challenge and learn to navigate its pitfalls. One might suggest, as Dr Rohrbaugh said, having "a structurally humble approach" that recognizes both the enormity of racism and one's need for help understanding its underpinnings.[31]

Conversely, early-career psychiatrists who take umbrage at the different perspective and seeming flippancy of our more seasoned colleagues might consider a different approach and instead recall our collective goal: equity for all, especially for our patients. While shunning powerful colleagues may feel good or validate one's individual position, it does not often move a movement structurally on its own. Structural racism can behave like the mythical Greek Hydra—cutting off its head may temporarily wound the beast, until more heads grow in its place. Accordingly, until we collectively acquire power and then choose to wield it toward justice, inequity will persist.

And who says that when today's young advocate-leaders find themselves at the helm, that they will not err, to the umbrage taken and chagrin of their junior peers? And were not those in power today, whose performance we lament, working hard to challenge the leadership that preceded them? Each generation must be humble, learn from predecessors, and understand that only decades from now our own flaws might forestall equity for the new generation.

CLINICS CARE POINTS

- Organizing psychiatrists potentiates impact
- To persuade, meet the audience where they stand and bring them toward your viewpoint
- Policy change often requires a persistent attention to detail
- Follow the money

DISCLOSURE

This project was supported by the Yale National Clinician Scholars Program and by CTSA Grant Number TL1 TR001864 from the National Center for Advancing Translational Science (NCATS), a component of the National Institutes of Health (NIH). Its contents are solely the responsibility of the authors and do not necessarily represent the official view of NIH. Dr. Mensah is Co-Editor of the Race and Mental Health Equity Column in Psychiatric Services. In 2020, he received a one-time speaking honoraria from the American Medical Association.

REFERENCES

1. Mensah MO, Ogbu-Nwobodo L, Shim RS. Racism and mental health equity: history repeating itself. Psychiatr Serv 2021;72(9):1091–4.
2. Stewart AJ. Dismantling structural racism in academic psychiatry to achieve workforce diversity. Am J Psychiatry 2021;178(3):210–2.
3. Sudak DM, Stewart AJ. Can we talk? the role of organized psychiatry in addressing structural racism to achieve diversity and inclusion in psychiatric workforce development. Acad Psychiatry 2021;45(1):89–92.
4. Jordan A, Shim RS, Rodriguez CI, et al. Psychiatry diversity leadership in academic medicine: guidelines for success. Am J Psychiatry 2021;178(3):224–8.
5. Bryant BE, Jordan A, Clark US. Race as a Social Construct in Psychiatry Research and Practice. JAMA Psychiatry 2022;79(2):93–4.
6. Mensah MO, Sommers BD. The policy argument for healthcare workforce diversity. J Gen Intern Med 2016;31(11):1369–72.
7. Marrast LM, Zallman L, Woolhandler S, et al. Minority physicians' role in the care of underserved patients: diversifying the physician workforce may be key in addressing health disparities. JAMA Intern Med 2014;174(2):289–91.

8. Busch SH, Ndumele CD, Loveridge CF, et al. Patient characteristics and treatment patterns among psychiatrists who do not accept private insurance. Psychiatr Serv 2019;70(1):35–9.

9. Bishop TF, Press MJ, Keyhani S, et al. Acceptance of insurance by psychiatrists and the implications for access to mental health care. JAMA Psychiatry 2014; 71(2 181).

10. Harris HW, Felder D, Clark MO. A psychiatric residency curriculum on the care of African American patients. Acad Psychiatry 2004;28(3):226–39.

11. Zatzick DF, Lu FG. The ethnic/minority focus unit as a training site in transcultural psychiatry. Acad Psychiatry 1991;15(4):218–25.

12. ACGME, ACfGME. Common program requirements (residency). ACGME approved major revision: June 10, 2018; effective: July 1, 2019. Accreditation Council for Graduate Medical Education (ACGME); 2019.

13. Mote J, Fulford D. Now is the time to support black individuals in the US living with serious mental illness—a call to action. JAMA Psychiatry 2021;78(2):129–30.

14. Metzl JM. The protest psychosis: how schizophrenia became a black disease. Beacon Press; 2010.

15. Bromberg W, Simon F. The protest psychosis: a special type of reactive psychosis. Arch Gen Psychiatry 1968;19(2):155–60.

16. Essien UR, Dusetzina SB, Gellad WF. A Policy Prescription for Reducing Health Disparities-Achieving Pharmacoequity. JAMA 2021;326(18):1793–4.

17. Hearne J, Grady A. Prescription Drug Coverage Under Medicaid. Congressional Information Service, Library of Congress; 2006.

18. Steele CM. Whistling Vivaldi: how stereotypes affect us and what we can do. WW Norton & Company; 2011.

19. Mensah MO. Majority taxes — toward antiracist allyship in medicine. New Engl J Med 2020;e23.

20. Cyrus KD. A piece of my mind: medical education and the minority tax. JAMA 2017;317(18):1833–4.

21. Association AP. The Principles of Medical Ethics With Annotations Especially Applicable to Psychiatry. American Journal of Psychiatry 1973;130(9):1057–64.

22. Stotland NL. Reproductive Rights and Women's Mental Health. Psychiatr Clin North Am 2017;40(2):335–50.

23. Stotland NL, Shrestha AD. More Evidence That Abortion Is Not Associated With Increased Risk of Mental Illness. JAMA Psychiatry 2018;75(8):775–6.

24. McGuire TG, Miranda J. New evidence regarding racial and ethnic disparities in mental health: policy implications. Health Aff (Project Hope) 2008;27(2):393–403.

25. Satcher DS. Executive summary: a report of the Surgeon General on mental health. Public Health Rep 2000;115(1):89–101.

26. Office of the Surgeon G, Center for Mental Health S, National Institute of Mental H. Publications and Reports of the Surgeon General. In: Mental health: culture, race, and ethnicity: a supplement to mental health: a Report of the Surgeon general. Rockville (MD): Substance Abuse and Mental Health Services Administration (US); 2001.

27. Henderson DC. Schizophrenia and comorbid metabolic disorders. J Clin Psychiatry 2005;66(Suppl 6):11–20.

28. Henderson DC. Metabolic Differences of Antipsychotics Among the Races. CNS Spectrums 2005;10(S2):13–20.

29. Henderson DC, Nguyen DD, Copeland PM, et al. Clozapine, diabetes mellitus, hyperlipidemia, and cardiovascular risks and mortality: results of a 10-year naturalistic study. J Clin Psychiatry 2005;66(9):1116–21.

30. Center BM. Health Equity Accelerator. Boston Medical Center. 2022. Avaialble at: https://www.bmc.org/health-equity-accelerator. Accessed February 28 2022.
31. Hansen H, Braslow J, Rohrbaugh RM. From Cultural to Structural Competency— Training Psychiatry Residents to Act on Social Determinants of Health and Institutional Racism. JAMA Psychiatry 2018;75(2):117–8.
32. Jenkins CD, Tuthill RW, Tannenbaum SI, et al. Zones of excess mortality in Massachusetts. New Engl J Med 1977;296(23):1354–6.
33. Black D. Inequalities in health. Report of a research working group. London: DHSS; 1980.
34. Statistics BoL. Occupational Outlook Handbook, Physicians and Surgeons. 2022. Available at: https://www.bls.gov/ooh/healthcare/physicians-and-surgeons.htm#tab-5.
35. Ung L, Stanford FC, Chodosh J. "All Labor Has Dignity" — The Case for Wage Equity for Essential Health Care Workers. New Engl J Med 2021;385(17): 1539–42.
36. Relman AS. Medical Professionalism in a Commercialized Health Care Market. JAMA 2007;298(22):2668–70.
37. Chen CL, Gold GJ, Cannesson M, et al. Calling Out Aversive Racism in Academic Medicine. New Engl J Med 2021;385(27):2499–501.
38. Sabshin M, Diesnhaus H, Wilkerson R. Dimensions of Institutional Racism in Psychiatry. Am J Psychiatry 1970;127(6):787–93.
39. Poussaint AF. Yes: it can be a delusional symptom of psychotic disorders. West J Med 2002;176(1):4.
40. Stewart AJ. Response to the Presidential Address. Am J Psychiatry 2018;175(8): 726–7.
41. McGhee H. The Sum of Us: What Racism Costs Everyone and How We Can Prosper Together. One World; 2021.
42. Barceló NE, Shadravan S. Race, Metaphor, and Myth in Academic Medicine. Academic Psychiatry; 2020. p. 1–6.

Workforce Diversity, Equity, and Inclusion

A Crucial Component of Professionalism in Psychiatry

Howard Y. Liu, MD, MBA[a,*], Allison R. Larson, MD, MS[b],
Sheritta A. Strong, MD[a], Ranna Parekh, MD, MPH[c],
Mamta Gautam, MD, MBA[d], Laura E. Flores, PhD[e],
Julie K. Silver, MD[f]

KEYWORDS

- Professionalism • Medical education • Workforce disparities • Psychiatry
- Medical professionalism

KEY POINTS

- Psychiatry has the opportunity to lead the medical workforce in incorporating diversity, equity, and inclusion into professionalism standards.
- Medical education would benefit from an expanded definition of professionalism to include workforce diversity, equity, and inclusion.
- Workforce disparities have negatively impacted the training and career advancement of many people, including but not limited to, individuals who identify with underrepresented racial and ethnic minority groups, women, people with disabilities, and the lesbian, gay, bisexual, transgender, and queer or questioning+ community.

This article originally appeared in *Psychiatric Clinics*, Volume 45 Issue 2, June 2022.

[a] University of Nebraska Medical Center, 985578 Nebraska Medical Center, Omaha, NE 68198-5578, USA; [b] Georgetown University, MedStar Washington Hospital Center, 5530 Wisconsin Ave, Suite 660, Chevy Chase, MD 20815, USA; [c] The University of Texas MD Anderson Cancer Center, 1515 Holcombe Boulevard, Houston, TX 77030, USA; [d] Psychosocial Oncology Program, The Ottawa Hospital Cancer Center, TOH General Campus, 501 Smyth Road, Ottawa, ON K1H 8L6, Canada; [e] College of Allied Health Professions, University of Nebraska Medical Center, 984035 Nebraska Medical Center, Omaha, NE 68198-4035, USA; [f] Department of Physical Medicine and Rehabilitation, Harvard Medical School, Massachusetts General Hospital, 55 Fruit Street, Boston, MA 02114 USA

* Corresponding author. UNMC Department of Psychiatry, 985575 Nebraska Medical Center, Omaha, NE 68198-5575.

E-mail address: hyliu@unmc.edu

Child Adolesc Psychiatric Clin N Am 33 (2024) 17–32
https://doi.org/10.1016/j.chc.2023.06.003
childpsych.theclinics.com

INTRODUCTION

Professionalism is an integral part of every aspect of medicine, and psychiatrists play a critical role in helping to frame discussions, didactics, and policy around this important topic. Indeed, for better or worse, DeJong[1] noted that psychiatrists are often held to a higher ethical standard than other physicians owing to the nature of their work. She conceptualized professionalism as one component of a Venn diagram with 3 overlapping concepts: professionalism, psychiatry, and the law. However, as Dingle and colleagues[2] point out, academic medical centers are "an environment in which there are a diversity of values, some of them contradictory or not obvious." Furthermore, there is a "hidden curriculum" in academia, which may cause ambiguity about core values and undermine psychological safety.[3]

Although professionalism definitions have evolved, there is no doubt that it is universally embraced in medicine (**Fig. 1**). Today, professionalism covers many topics ranging from research misconduct to social media behaviors, and in this report, the authors focus on *workforce diversity, equity, and inclusion* (DEI)—an often-neglected topic in professionalism literature, training, and discussions. Although women now outnumber men matriculating into medical schools in the United States, Canada, and many European Union countries, racial and ethnic diversification of the physician workforce is moving slowly.[4] Similarly, the proportion of people identifying with an underrepresented group (eg, racial/ethnic, lesbian, gay, bisexual, transgender, and queer or questioning+ [LGBTQ+], disability) or being at the intersection of multiple historically or socially marginalized groups is increasing in most specialties, including psychiatry, but the growth remains slow.

There is a growing body of literature that demonstrates many forms of bias have a profound impact on academic medicine and training and working environments. The Association of American Medical Colleges (AAMC) announced a new initiative that is focused on gender equity and included "workforce" as one of 4 areas of emphasis, along with leadership/compensation, research, and recognition.[5] The AAMC stated, "Gender equity is a key factor in achieving excellence in medicine." Of course, one should strive for equity for the entire workforce regardless of gender. Importantly,

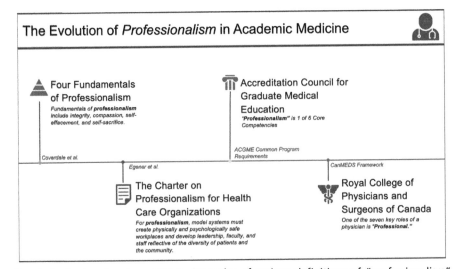

Fig. 1. Professionalism in medicine. Examples of various definitions of "professionalism" used among medical education researchers and medical training organizations.

all forms of bias affect not only those who are targeted but also bystanders and patients.

Thus, the authors turn their lens to physician workforce DEI as a crucial, but often neglected, component of professionalism.[6–8] Professionalism conventionally includes several important topics that specifically concern psychiatrists, including patient care disparities, research conflict-of-interest disclosures, academic productivity and leadership, and physician wellness. The authors aim to highlight the value of including workforce DEI as a crucial component of professionalism. Although this applies to the entire workforce, the focus is on physicians and more specifically the field of psychiatry. This report addresses various barriers and strategies for addressing workforce DEI in psychiatry, some of which are shown in **Fig. 2**.

THE EVOLUTION OF PROFESSIONALISM IN ACADEMIC MEDICINE

Historically, there are numerous definitions of professionalism in academic medicine and psychiatry. As Roberts and colleagues noted,[9] professionalism definitions differ in emphasizing ideals, obligations, virtues, attitudes, and ethical practices. Coverdale and colleagues[10] focused on the importance of "four fundamental virtues of integrity, compassion, self-effacement, and self-sacrifice in the teaching of ethics and professionalism." These virtues were traced back to the published work of Dr. John Gregory of Scotland (1724–1773), who called on physicians to serve as the moral fiduciary of the patient and place the needs of the patient above their self-interest.

In 2017, Egener and colleagues[6] included The Charter on Professionalism for Health Care Organizations (HCOs) that discussed commitments to a healthy workplace and inclusion and diversity within the organizational culture. To nurture professionalism, encourage the pursuit of employee excellence, and achieve outstanding health care with the broader community, The Charter on Professionalism suggested that model HCOs create workplace environments that are physically and psychologically safe, and foster development of leadership, faculty, and staff members that are reflective of the diversity of patients and the community. The Accreditation Council for Graduate

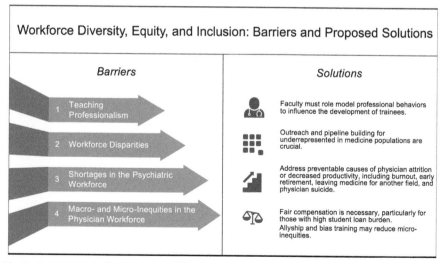

Fig. 2. Barriers and solutions to workforce DEI. Some of the barriers to increasing workforce DEI and proposed solutions for each barrier.

Medical Education (ACGME) has made professionalism one of its 6 core competencies (**Box 1**), and this is now integrated into residency milestones. The ACGME expects faculty members who train residents to be exemplars of professionalism and evaluates both faculty and residency programs on their professionalism development programs.[11] Similarly, in Canada, the Royal College of Physicians and Surgeons of Canada offers the CanMEDS framework that identifies and describes the abilities physicians require to effectively meet the health care needs of the people they serve.[12] One of the 7 key roles of a physician is Professional, noting that physicians are committed to the health and well-being of individual patients and society through ethical practice, high personal standards of behavior, accountability to the profession and society, physician-led regulation, and maintenance of personal health.

Despite different frames of professionalism, there is a consensus that professionalism must be cultivated, assessed, and refined in practice. As Roberts[13] stated, it is imperative to "see how these exquisite ideals about the roles and obligations of physicians translate in real life—with its uncertainties, unexpected complexities, and unjust cruelties—into clear prescriptions for honorable conduct and ethically sound decision making." On the contrary, Schwartz and colleagues[14] emphasized that, "teaching professionalism as a theoretical subject will likely have little influence upon the behavior of future physicians." Instead, faculty must role model professional behaviors to influence the development of trainees. A study of 3 psychiatry residency programs noted, when residents are assessed by the Clinical Competency Committee biannually, it is critical to maximize the number of end-of-rotation assessments to improve reliability.[15] In other words, more eyes on the trainees lead to a better assessment of clinical performance, including professionalism. Emphasizing the importance of continued professionalism training, Silver and colleagues[4] wrote that this ethical commitment must continue throughout the physician's career. "Although ethics principles can be taught, it is incumbent upon the individual to have an internal sense of responsibility and a commitment to 'doing the right thing' while achieving the best possible outcome for every patient."

PHYSICIAN DISPARITIES AND PATIENT CARE

Focusing on patient care disparities is an important component of professionalism and is well documented in the literature describing professionalism; in juxtaposition, workforce disparities that can impact patient care disparities have received far less consideration.[7] A recent review published in the journal *Health Equity* titled "Physician

---

Box 1
American College of Graduate Medical Education core competencies

Professionalism

Patient care

Medical knowledge

Practice-based learning & improvement

Interpersonal & communication skills

Systems-based practice

Professionalism is one of 6 ACGME core competencies. Each competency is made up of milestones that trainees are required to master at key stages of their medical training.

Workforce Disparities and Patient Care: A Narrative Review" focused on the role and impact of workforce disparities on patient care.[4] This review highlighted many important issues briefly described here. Equitable inclusion of the physician workforce is often measured as a reflection of the evolving demographics in the United States and other countries. Many medical schools' workforce diversity strategies are heavily focused on the recruitment of people who identify with racial and/or ethnic minority groups and are underrepresented in medicine (URiM), as a workforce that is reflective of the population may be a key component to reducing health care disparities.

Some studies suggest that women physicians are more likely to care for female patients and may spend more time discussing preventative medicine or have unique insights regarding symptoms (eg, cardiac symptoms).[16] Similarly, URiM physicians more often practice primary care and return to their communities to care for patients from underrepresented racial/ethnic groups, compared with their non-URiM peers.[4] There is evidence to suggest that people who identify with ethnic/racial minority groups may prefer physicians who have a similar demographic background,[17] and in some cases, such as Black infant mortality, racial concordance may positively affect outcomes.[18]

As these issues are inextricably linked, there is an urgent need to address workforce and patient care disparities simultaneously by including DEI as a core competency of professionalism.

DEVELOPING AND SUPPORTING A STRONG PSYCHIATRY WORKFORCE

Developing and supporting the strongest possible psychiatry workforce means encouraging medical students to enter the specialty and decreasing attrition at every stage of their careers (**Fig. 3**). Indeed, the psychiatric workforce needs shoring up, as there are current and predicted shortages across the United States. Between 2003 and 2013, there was a 0.2% decrease in the absolute number of practicing psychiatrists in the United States and a population adjusted-mean decline of nearly 10%.[19] The Health Resources and Services Administration analyzed 2016 data, anticipating

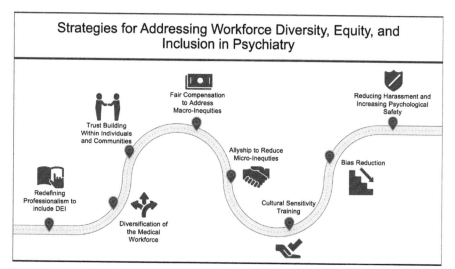

Fig. 3. Strategies for addressing workforce DEI in psychiatry. These are examples of strategies for addressing and increasing workforce DEI in the field of psychiatry.

that by 2030 there will be a shortage of 4820 to 7810 full-time equivalents (FTE) of adult psychiatrists and a shortage of 680 to 1240 FTE of child and adolescent psychiatrists.[20] The psychiatric workforce shortage reflects data describing total physician workforce shortages, highlighting a need both within and outside of psychiatry.[21]

Disability is an important part of DEI, and students with mental health conditions and/or physical disabilities may require additional support and reasonable accommodations.[22] Learners with disabilities who enter psychiatry practice may have unique perspectives and help to close gaps for patients who have disabilities.

Similarly, adoption of policies and practices for LGBTQ+ learners is crucial in the commitment to DEI, and for the optimal care of patients. It is well documented that systemic practices in medicine are alienating to LGBTQ+ patients and physicians alike, and that many learners continue to conceal their identity for fear of harassment and discrimination.[23] This is yet another opportunity for communities with unique perspectives to feel safe in their learning environment, close gaps with patients, and provide a necessary perspective to the medical system as a whole.

In academic medicine, the leaky pipeline for women and URiM individuals is well documented, with women less likely to advance to leadership positions[24] and more likely to drop out of certain residency training programs.[25] In addition, resident physicians from URiM groups are more likely to report additional burdens during residency training because of their racial or ethnic status.[26]

To address the current and future psychiatric workforce shortages, there needs to be more people pursuing, entering, and remaining in the field. This will require addressing factors including burnout, early retirement, leaving medicine for another field, suicide, and so forth.[19,27] That is to say, it is crucial to address *preventable* causes of physician attrition or decreased productivity.

ADDRESSING MACROINEQUITIES IN THE PHYSICIAN WORKFORCE

Although there are many documented inequities contributing to disparities in the psychiatric workforce, ensuring fair compensation is among the most critically important to address. Research studies and national surveys have consistently found that compensation disparities exist based on gender and race.[28–33] Ly and colleagues[30] compared salaries within a multispecialty cohort of physicians and found that Black men received similar salaries to White women, which were less than White men and more than Black women. Multiple large United States studies have shown that gender-based differences in pay persist after adjustment for confounding factors, such as hours worked, years in practice, academic rank, practice type, specialty, geographic location, parental status, marital status, Medicare revenue, and National Institutes of Health (NIH) funding (**Table 1**).[24–29] Jena and colleagues[31] conducted a large-scale study of academic physicians in multiple specialties, including 455 psychiatrists. Psychiatry ranked 12th largest out of 18 specialties in terms of the magnitude of gender pay gap. A multivariable analysis was conducted, which took into account the following covariates: age, years of experience, NIH funding, publication count, clinical trial participation, Medicare payments, and medical school fixed effects. A difference in salary of $14,799 (95% confidence interval = −$5709 to $35,308) existed between the men (n = 294) and women (n = 161) psychiatrists, although this did not reach significance. A similar salary gap was found in the psychiatry subspecialty of psychosomatic medicine, with Rosenthal and Sabuco[34] reporting a significant (nonadjusted) mean salary difference of $20,000 between men and women. According to 2017 AAMC data, the gender compensation gap in US psychiatry was the sixth greatest out of 28 departments: women made $0.81 for every $1 made by men.[35]

Table 1
Examples of compensation studies in psychiatry[a4-7,28,29,36]

Authors	Source	Participants (Total N)	Confounding Variables	Gender Salary Gap (Disparities Are in Favor of Men in all Studies with Gaps)
Research studies				
Jagsi et al[1]	Physician researchers who have received K08 or K23 NIH funding	Physician-researchers (800)	Age, race, marital status, parental status, additional graduate degrees, academic rank, leadership positions, specialty	$12,194
Nguyen Le et al[2]	Integrated Public Use Microdata Series census and 5-y American Community Survey sample for 2007–2011	Physicians (113,586)	Age, number of children, hours worked per week, race, marital status, self-employment status, weeks worked per year	$51,100
Steffler et al[3]	Ontario (Canada) Health Insurance Plan	Physicians (31,481; 2202 psychiatrists)	Tenure, part-time status, after-hours work, holiday work, weekend work, primary care payment model, practice setting, academic physician status, rurality	No salary gap after adjustment
Ly et al[4]	US Census American Community Survey	Physicians (61,327; 938 psychiatrists)	Hours worked, years in practice, practice type, specialty type, state of residence, time period, percentage revenue from Medicare/Medicaid	$85,921

(continued on next page)

Table 1
(continued)

Authors	Source	Participants (Total N)	Confounding Variables	Gender Salary Gap (*Disparities Are in Favor of Men in all Studies with Gaps*)
Jena et al[5]	Published salary data of physicians at 24 publicly funded medical schools	Physicians in academia (10,241;455 psychiatrists)	Age, years of experience, faculty rank, specialty, scientific authorship, NIH funding, clinical trial participation, Medicare reimbursements	$19,878
National physician surveys				
Medscape[6]	National physician survey of Medscape members	US psychiatrists (approximately 1074)	Unadjusted	$49,000
Doximity[7]	National physician survey	US full-time physicians (approximately 135,000)	Unadjusted	$116,000

Numerous studies have demonstrated pay gaps for women in medicine, and the reports highlighted in this table summarize some of the findings that are relevant to psychiatry. Importantly, many of these studies account for confounding variables, and thus the pay gaps are typically attributed to gender-related bias.
[a] This is not intended to be a complete list of compensation studies.

Gender disparities in pay are not limited to the United States. Steffler and colleagues[36] conducted a robust study reporting on 99% of the physician workforce in Ontario, Canada (n = 31,481). A significant unadjusted pay gap of 17% was found by gender for the 2202 psychiatrists included in this study; however, the gap became nonsignificant after adjusting for tenure, part-time status, after-hours work, weekend work, primary care payment model, practice setting, academic physician status, and rurality.

Numerous institutions have instituted successful programs to combat compensation disparities through data collection and monitoring, building multivariable models for data analysis, identifying systems-level barriers and individual outliers, and working closely with department chairs to correct identified disparities.[35,37]

In addition to frank pay disparities, variation in student loan burden contributes to workforce disparities, particularly among URiM and first-generation physicians. The connection between the magnitude of student loan debt and specialty choice has been well studied; students carrying greater debt are more likely to select higher-paying specialties.[38] In Medscape's 2021 Physician Compensation Report, psychiatry was the eighth lowest compensated specialty out of the 29 reported, with only 69% of the psychiatrists reporting they felt fairly compensated. Despite this, of the 84% who would choose medicine again, 86% would choose psychiatry again, metrics that all fell within the top half of specialties.[32] In Doximity's 2020 Compensation Report, psychiatry was the 10th lowest compensated specialty.[33] Medical students who chose to specialize in psychiatry, on average, reported being less influenced by salary expectations and student loan debt compared with students who chose controllable lifestyle or surgical specialties, according to AAMC data.[39] However, compensation and debt impact recruitment into psychiatry as well as financial stress down the line.

The female-dominated subspecialty of child and adolescent psychiatry is an example of a subspecialty with comparatively low compensation and high debt burden. Many child and adolescent psychiatry fellows and early career attending physicians carry substantial educational debt.[36] Mann and colleagues[40] reported nearly half of their survey respondents owed more than $150,000 in student loans and anticipated full-time salaries between $175,000 and $250,000 following fellowship. A connection has been well described between high levels of debt and stress related to finances.[38] These salary disparities, when combined with educational debt, amplify financial stress for people entering this field, disproportionately harming women who make up a majority of child and adolescent psychiatrists.

Beyond compensation, there are numerous other macroinequities in psychiatry that have been documented for women and people who identify with an underrepresented group. For example, women are underrepresented on journal editorial boards[41] and as plenary/keynote speakers at major society conferences.[42] These inequities can be swiftly corrected by including a proportional representation of women on conference committees and by continuing to invite women speakers and editorial board members if initial invitees decline. According to the AAMC academic psychiatry data, the percentage of women full-time MD faculty decreased from 53% of instructors to 20% of full professors in 2015.[43] Similarly, the percentage of people who identify with an underrepresented racial or ethnic group in medicine remained low in psychiatry for both men and women, peaking at the assistant professor level at 9.1% and falling to 5.4% at the full professor level.[43] Of permanent department chairs, 13.7% were women and 9.9% were people who identify with an underrepresented racial or ethnic group in 2015.[43] The percentage of women chairs increased to 22.1% in 2018, signaling an increase, while emphasizing a need for focus on gender equity in psychiatry leadership.[43]

Correction of these disparities involves a multifactorial approach that includes addressing systemic inequities, and the contributors to them, such as structural racism, in the promotional process, authorship, research funding, recognition awards, speaker invitations, and leadership positions. There are also interpersonal issues including, but not limited to, implicit bias.

ADDRESSING MICROINEQUITIES IN THE PHYSICIAN WORKFORCE

Microaggressions and microinequities are barriers to developing a strong and equitable workforce.[44] The term microaggression was first defined in 1969 by Harvard psychiatrist, Chester Pierce, MD, who used it to describe ephemeral indignities that conveyed hostility toward African Americans in the Jim Crowe era. The term has evolved to include persons from any community that have been marginalized or any person viewed as the "other."[45] Economist and former Massachusetts Institute of Technology professor Mary Rowe, PhD, coined the term microinequities to characterize a wider set of workplace harmful events that undermine workers who identified with at least one underrepresented group.[44] Cumulative microaggressions and microinequities result in an erosion of confidence in the learning environment, which can increase attrition among all groups at risk to leave.

As Sukhera[45] notes, "we are all both victim and perpetrator, and none of us are immune. Therefore, change starts with looking in the mirror; not by pointing our finger." The need for ongoing training is borne out by emerging studies that show differences in perception of implicit bias. One study exposed 124 faculty at 4 academic medical centers to videos depicting gender-based microaggressions and found that women faculty reported much higher frequencies of microaggressions than male faculty.[46]

One strategy to address the negative impact of microaggressions, Molina and colleagues[47] argues, is a deliberate attempt to foster microaffirmations, defined as "small acts, which are often ephemeral and hard-to-see, often unconscious efforts to help others succeed." Examples include appreciative inquiry, active listening, rewarding positive behaviors, intentional inclusion in professional meetings and networks, introducing team members by formal title, and being mindful of diverse representation in public spaces, such as portrait walls near lecture halls. In medical education, microaggressions, microinequities, and implicit bias are being incorporated into curricula to help students understand the effect on health and workforce outcomes and to provide strategies to improve the environment for everyone, particularly individuals who often experience implicit bias. Addressing microinequities in the workforce will also require consideration of cultural sensitivity training and development of cultural humility. This will enhance the ability of trainees to understand and respond effectively to others' cultural needs and to establish interpersonal relationships bridging cultural differences.

RECOGNIZING THE ROLE OF BIAS IN PHYSICIAN WORKFORCE DISPARITIES

Although there are many published studies documenting physician workforce disparities, the underlying causes are complex and generally multifactorial. Various forms of bias typically play a role in workforce disparities. Unfortunately, there are many examples of explicit (conscious) bias and structural discrimination in medicine. These are profoundly disturbing and require strategic and systemic changes.

A more common cause of physician workforce disparities is implicit (unconscious) bias, although rooting out implicit bias is challenging because it is not intentional or conscious. Numerous studies have documented troubling patterns of implicit bias impacting URiM students as early as medical school.[48] This trend continues into residency training with one study of United States resident physicians identifying gender bias favoring men in leadership positions.[49] Continued implicit bias through training and even into medical careers results in lower work satisfaction for URiM physicians.[48] Furthermore, implicit bias appears to be associated with symptoms of burnout that begin early in training.[4,50]

Another form of bias is *structural*, and this is likely a factor in physician workforce disparities. Structural bias stems from the term, "structural racism," which is defined as the macrolevel systems, social forces, institutions, ideologies, and processes that interact with one another to generate and reinforce inequities among racial and ethnic groups.[51] When applied to the physician workforce, structural bias may have ramifications on what groups of people have access to the resources needed to pursue medical training[52] and who can succeed in medical training. Furthermore, the closing of historically Black medical schools owing to the Flexner report has resulted in an estimated loss of more than 30,000 Black physicians.[53]

THE ROLE OF ALLIES

Allies have an increasingly vital role in ensuring the medical workplace is safe, and in mitigating macroinequities and microinequities. An ally is any person who supports, empowers, or stands up for another person or a group of people. Allyship involves a person from a nonmarginalized group, an ally, who uses their privilege to advocate for those from historically or socially marginalized groups. Medical leaders should take personal responsibility for their own attitudes and behaviors, support and promote women colleagues, and view allyship as a strategic mechanism to fight injustice and promote equity and inclusion.[54] An example of a leadership strategy to incorporate DEI as a valued competency within psychiatry might be the recognition of DEI activity as scholarly work. This may help move the needle for those who identify with underrepresented groups as they often perform disproportionately more DEI work, with little recognition toward promotion.

REDUCING HARASSMENT AND INCREASING PSYCHOLOGICAL SAFETY

In 2018, the National Academies of Science, Engineering, and Medicine released a report titled "Sexual Harassment of Women: Climate, Culture, and Consequences in Academic Sciences, Engineering, and Medicine."[55] The report acknowledged there has been more research, activity, and funding aimed at improving the recruitment, retention, and advancement of women; although this has led to more women entering these fields, women continue to face many biases and barriers, including sexual harassment and racial/ethnic harassment.[56] Sexual harassment in academia has been shown to negatively impact the recruitment, retention, and advancement of women, and the report provided 15 key recommendations for the future. Nembhard and Edmondson[57] have described the concept of psychological safety in the workplace, and how to create a culture in which people feel valued, recognized, respected, and supported.

DECREASING BURNOUT AND IMPROVING WELLNESS

Burnout is a pervasive problem in the psychiatry workforce and is multifactorial. Although bias is often unintentional, the consequences can be serious and have been linked to poor physician health in the literature. For example, in the 2017 Canadian Medical Association survey, women physicians reported significantly higher rates of burnout, depression, and suicidal ideation than men.[58] Dissatisfaction with work-life integration predicted a 3 times greater likelihood of burnout; dissatisfaction with their career in medicine led to a ninefold increase in the likelihood of burnout. Dissatisfaction with careers can result from discrimination, which includes disparaging or disrespectful treatment or comments; lack of career promotion; and disparities in resources (including financial and administrative support), rewards, and reimbursement.[59] Women who belong to underrepresented racial or ethnic groups and have intersectional identities may face additional and even exponential discrimination, which can impact their sense of well-being, belonging, and perception of workplace stress. Experts recognize that unless these factors are addressed effectively by health care organizations, women physicians will continue to be at high risk for burnout.[60,61] In addition to the cost of burnout to the individual physician, negative impact on their clinical care, and poor organizational outcomes, there is also a significant financial cost related to physician turnover and reduced clinical hours attributable to burnout each year in the United States.[61–64] Addressing these inequities is imperative to ensure the wellness of the medical profession.

SUMMARY

This report aims to encourage the adoption of workforce DEI as a crucial component of professionalism. Historically and socially marginalized students, trainees, and practicing physicians face many barriers throughout their careers, and this report highlights opportunities for the specialty of psychiatry to better address them. Psychiatry has always been a leader in understanding the role of diversity in medicine and the need for organized advocacy. This historical context suggests that psychiatrists are well positioned to endorse incorporating workforce DEI as a standard part of professionalism.

COMPLIANCE WITH ETHICAL STANDARDS

The authors have reviewed the journal's ethical standards and attest to their compliance with these standards in this submission.

ETHICAL CONSIDERATIONS

N/A.

FUNDING SOURCES

None.

ACKNOWLEDGMENTS

The authors wish to thank leaders across all health care institutions who are championing diversity, equity, and inclusion for the future of our workforce in psychiatry and medicine.

DISCLOSURE

H.Y. Liu reports no disclosures related to this work. Unrelated to this work, Dr Liu receives honoraria and travel support as a member of the National Advisory Council for the Robert Wood Johnson Foundation's Clinical Scholars Program, receives travel support as a Counselor for the Association of Directors of Medical Student Education in Psychiatry, has received honoraria from Elsevier for serving as a guest editor, has received travel support and honoraria for invited talks, such as Grand Rounds lectures. A.R. Larson reports no disclosures related to this work. Unrelated to this work, Dr Larson has served on a one-time advisory board for Sanofi Genzyme on resident education and has received honoraria for invited lectures such as medical conference and Grand Rounds lectures. S.A. Strong reports no disclosures related to or unrelated to this work. R. Parekh reports no disclosures related to this work. Unrelated to this work, Dr Parekh has published books and receives royalties from book publishers, and she gives professional talks such as grand rounds and medical conference lectures and receives honoraria from conference organizers. M. Gautam reports no disclosures related to this work. Unrelated to this work, Dr Gautam is CEO of PEAK MD Inc, through which she receives fees for academic grand rounds and conference keynote presentations, medical leadership development, health care consulting, coaching physician leaders. L.E. Flores reports no disclosures related to this work. J.K. Silver reports no disclosures related to this work. Unrelated to this work, as an academic physician, Dr Silver has published books and receives royalties from book publishers, and she gives professional talks such as grand rounds and medical conference plenary lectures and receives honoraria from conference organizers. She is a venture partner in Third Culture Capital and has participated in research funded by the Binational Scientific Foundation.

REFERENCES

1. DeJong SM. Professionalism and technology: competencies across the tele-behavioral health and E-behavioral health spectrum. Acad Psychiatry 2018; 42(6):800–7.
2. Dingle A, DeJong S, Madaan V, et al. Teaching ethics in child and adolescent psychiatry: vignette-based curriculum. MedEdPORTAL 2016;12:10418.
3. Torralba KD, Jose D, Byrne J. Psychological safety, the hidden curriculum, and ambiguity in medicine. Clin Rheumatol 2020;39(3):667–71.
4. Silver JK, Bean AC, Slocum C, et al. Physician workforce disparities and patient care: a narrative review. Health equity 2019;3(1):360–77.
5. Association of American Medical Colleges A. Gender equity in academic medicine. AAMC Board of Directors. 2021. Available at: https://www.aamc.org/news-insights/gender-equity-academic-medicine. Accessed November 6, 2021.
6. Egener BE, Mason DJ, McDonald WJ, et al. The charter on professionalism for health care organizations. Acad Med 2017;92(8):1091–9.
7. Silver JK, Cuccurullo S, Weiss LD, et al. The vital role of professionalism in physical medicine and rehabilitation. Am J Phys Med Rehabil 2020;99(4):273–7.
8. Erdahl LM, Chandrabose RK, Pitt SC, et al. A call for professionalism: addressing gender bias in surgical training. J Surg Educ 2020;77(4):718–9.
9. Weiss Roberts L, Coverdale J, Louie A. Professionalism and the ethics-related roles of academic psychiatrists. Acad Psychiatry 2005;29(5):413–5.
10. Coverdale JH, Balon R, Roberts LW. Cultivating the professional virtues in medical training and practice. Acad Psychiatry 2011;35(3):155–9.
11. Accreditation Council for Graduate Medical Education A. ACGME common program requirements (residency). ACGME. Nov. 6, 2021, 2021. 2021. Available at: https://www.acgme.org/globalassets/PFAssets/ProgramRequirements/CPRResidency2021.pdf. Accessed November 6, 2021.
12. Canada RCoPaSo. CanMEDS: better standards, better physicians, better care. Royal College of Physicians and Surgeons of Canada. Nov. 6, 2021, 2021. 2021. Available at: https://www.royalcollege.ca/rcsite/canmeds/canmeds-framework-e. Accessed November 6, 2021.

13. Roberts LW. Professionalism in psychiatry: a very special collection. Acad Psychiatry 2009;33(6):429–30.
14. Schwartz AC, Kotwicki RJ, McDonald WM. Developing a modern standard to define and assess professionalism in trainees. Acad Psychiatry 2009;33(6):442–50.
15. Lloyd RB, Park YS, Tekian A, et al. Understanding assessment systems for clinical competency committee decisions: evidence from a multisite study of psychiatry residency training programs. Acad Psychiatry 2020;44(6):734–40.
16. Nakayama A, Morita H, Fujiwara T, et al. Effect of treatment by female cardiologists on short-term readmission rates of patients hospitalized with cardiovascular diseases. Circ J 2019;83(9):1937–43.
17. Takeshita J, Wang S, Loren AW, et al. Association of racial/ethnic and gender concordance between patients and physicians with patient experience ratings. JAMA Netw Open 2020;3(11):e2024583.
18. Greenwood BN, Hardeman RR, Huang L, et al. Physician-patient racial concordance and disparities in birthing mortality for newborns. Proc Natl Acad Sci U S A 2020;117(35):21194–200.
19. Bishop TF, Seirup JK, Pincus HA, et al. Population of US practicing psychiatrists declined, 2003-13, which may help explain poor access to mental health care. Health Aff (Project Hope) 2016;35(7):1271–7.
20. U.S Department of Health and Human Services Health Resources and Services Administration; Bureau of Health Workforce NCfHWA. State-level projections of supply and demand for behavioral health occupations: 2016-2030. Nov.6, 2021, 2021. 2021. Available at: https://bhw.hrsa.gov/sites/default/files/bureau-health-workforce/data-research/state-level-estimates-report-2018.pdf. Accessed November 6, 2021.
21. Association of American Medical Colleges A. The complexities of physician supply and demand: projections from 2018 to 2033. AAMC. Nov. 6, 2021, 2021. 2021. Available at: https://www.aamc.org/system/files/2020-06/stratcomm-aamc-physician-workforce-projections-june-2020.pdf. Accessed November 6, 2021.
22. Golden RN, Petty EM. Learners with disabilities: an important component of diversity, equity, and inclusion in medical education. Acad Med 2021. https://doi.org/10.1097/ACM.0000000000004496.
23. Mansh M, White W, Gee-Tong L, et al. Sexual and gender minority identity disclosure during undergraduate medical education: "in the closet" in medical school. Acad Med 2015;90(5):634–44.
24. Lewiss RE, Silver JK, Bernstein CA, et al. Is academic medicine making mid-career women physicians invisible? J Womens Health (Larchmt) 2020;29(2):187–92.
25. Yeo HL, Abelson JS, Symer MM, et al. Association of time to attrition in surgical residency with individual resident and programmatic factors. JAMA Surg 2018;153(6):511–7.
26. Osseo-Asare A, Balasuriya L, Huot SJ, et al. Minority resident physicians' views on the role of race/ethnicity in their training experiences in the workplace. JAMA Netw Open 2018;1(5):e182723.
27. McFarland DC, Hlubocky F, Riba M. Update on addressing mental health and burnout in physicians: what is the role for psychiatry? Curr Psychiatry Rep 2019;21(11):108.
28. Jagsi R, Griffith KA, Stewart A, et al. Gender differences in the salaries of physician researchers. JAMA 2012;307(22):2410–7.

29. Nguyen Le TA, Lo Sasso AT, Vujicic M. Trends in the earnings gender gap among dentists, physicians, and lawyers. J Am Dent Assoc 2017;148(4):257–62.e2.

30. Ly DP, Seabury SA, Jena AB. Differences in incomes of physicians in the United States by race and sex: observational study. BMJ 2016;353:i2923.

31. Jena AB, Olenski AR, Blumenthal DM. Sex differences in physician salary in US public medical schools. JAMA Intern Med 2016;176(9):1294–304.

32. Martin K. Medscape psychiatrist compensation report 2021. Medscape. Nov. 6, 2021, 2021. 2021. Available at: https://www.medscape.com/slideshow/2021-compensation-psychiatrist-6013867. Accessed November 6, 2021.

33. Doximity. 2020 physician compensation report. Doximity, Inc. Nov. 6, 2021, 2021. 2021. Available at: https://www.doximity.com/2020_compensation_report. Accessed November 6, 2021.

34. Rosenthal LJ, Sabuco JJ. Salaries in psychosomatic medicine: a cross-sectional survey of practicing physicians. Psychosomatics 2017;58(1):92–4.

35. Dandar VMLD, Garrison GE. Promising practices for understanding and addressing salary equity at U.S. medical schools. Nov. 6, 2021, 2021. 2021. Available at: https://store.aamc.org/promising-practices-for-understanding-and-addressing-faculty-salary-equity-at-u-s-medical-schools.html. Accessed November 6, 2021.

36. Steffler M, Chami N, Hill S, et al. Disparities in physician compensation by gender in Ontario, Canada. JAMA Netw Open 2021;4(9):e2126107.

37. Hayes SN, Noseworthy JH, Farrugia G. A structured compensation plan results in equitable physician compensation: a single-center analysis. Mayo Clin Proc 2020;95(1):35–43.

38. Pisaniello MS, Asahina AT, Bacchi S, et al. Effect of medical student debt on mental health, academic performance and specialty choice: a systematic review. BMJ Open 2019;9(7):e029980.

39. Wilbanks L, Spollen J, Messias E. Factors influencing medical school graduates toward a career in psychiatry: analysis from the 2011-2013 Association of American Medical Colleges Graduation Questionnaire. Acad Psychiatry 2016;40(2):255–60.

40. Mann A, Tarshis T, Joshi SV. An exploratory survey of career choice, training, and practice trends in early career child and adolescent psychiatrists and fellows. Acad Psychiatry 2020. https://doi.org/10.1007/s40596-019-01167-y.

41. Hafeez DM, Waqas A, Majeed S, et al. Gender distribution in psychiatry journals' editorial boards worldwide. Compr Psychiatry 2019;94:152119.

42. Larson AR, Sharkey KM, Poorman JA, et al. Representation of women among invited speakers at medical specialty conferences. J Womens Health (Larchmt) 2020;29(4):550–60.

43. Association of American Medical Colleges A. The state of women in academic medicine. Nov. 6, 2021, 2021. 2021. Available at: https://www.aamc.org/data-reports/faculty-institutions/report/state-women-academic-medicine. Accessed November 6, 2021.

44. Silver JK, Rowe M, Sinha MS, et al. Micro-inequities in medicine. PM R 2018;10(10):1106–14.

45. Sukhera J. Breaking microaggressions without breaking ourselves. Perspect Med Education 2019;8(3):129–30.

46. Periyakoil VS, Chaudron L, Hill EV, et al. Common types of gender-based micro-aggressions in medicine. Acad Med 2020;95(3):450–7.

47. Molina RL, Ricciotti H, Chie L, et al. Creating a culture of micro-affirmations to overcome gender-based micro-inequities in academic medicine. Am J Med 2019;132(7):785–7.

48. Lawrence JA, Davis BA, Corbette T, et al. Racial/ethnic differences in burnout: a systematic review. J Racial Ethnic Health Disparities 2021. https://doi.org/10.1007/s40615-020-00950-0.
49. Hansen M, Schoonover A, Skarica B, et al. Implicit gender bias among US resident physicians. BMC Med Educ 2019;19(1):396.
50. Dyrbye L, Herrin J, West CP, et al. Association of racial bias with burnout among resident physicians. JAMA Netw Open 2019;2(7):e197457.
51. Powell JA. Structural racism: building upon the insights of John Calmore. North Carol Law Rev 2007;86:791.
52. Lucey CR, Saguil A. The consequences of structural racism on MCAT scores and medical school admissions: the past is prologue. Acad Med 2020;95(3):351–6.
53. Campbell KM, Corral I, Infante Linares JL, et al. Projected estimates of African American medical graduates of closed historically black medical schools. JAMA Netw Open 2020;3(8):e2015220.
54. Melaku TM, Angie B, Smith David G, et al. Be a better ally. Nov. 6, 2021, 2021. 2021. Available at: https://hbr.org/2020/11/be-a-better-ally. Accessed November 6, 2021.
55. National Academies of Sciences, Engineering, and Medicine 2018. Sexual Harassment of Women: Climate, Culture, and Consequences in Academic Sciences, Engineering, and Medicine. Washington, DC: The National Academies Press. https://doi.org/10.17226/24994.
56. Corbie-Smith G, Frank E, Nickens HW, et al. Prevalences and correlates of ethnic harassment in the U.S. Women Physicians' Health Study. Acad Med 1999;74(6):695–701.
57. Nembhard IM, Edmondson AC. Making it safe: the effects of leader inclusiveness and professional status on psychological safety and improvement efforts in health care teams. Journal of Organizational Behavior 2006;27(7):941–66.
58. Puddester D. The Canadian Medical Association's policy on physician health and well-being. West J Med 2001;174(1):5–7.
59. Templeton K, Bernstein CA, Sukhera J, et al. Gender-based differences in burnout: Issues faced by women physicians. NAM Perspectives. Discussion Paper, National Academy of Medicine, Washington, DC. https://doi.org/10.31478/201905a.
60. Shanafelt TD, Noseworthy JH. Executive leadership and physician well-being: nine organizational strategies to promote engagement and reduce burnout. Mayo Clin Proc 2017;92(1):129–46.
61. Chin EL, Britto VM, Parekh R. Diversity and medical professionalism. Health Aff Millwood 2020;39(4):722.
62. Canadian Medical Association C. Addressing gender equity and diversity in Canada's medical profession: a review. Federation of Medical Women of Canada. Nov. 6, 2021, 2021. 2021. Available at: https://www.cma.ca/sites/default/files/pdf/Ethics/report-2018-equity-diversity-medicine-e.pdf. Accessed November 6, 2021.
63. Han S, Shanafelt TD, Sinsky CA, et al. Estimating the attributable cost of physician burnout in the United States. Ann Intern Med 2019;170(11):784–90.
64. Rider EA, Diekman S, Doshi TL, et al. Answering the challenge: diversity, equity, and inclusion as a key to professionalism. Am J Med 2020;133(6):e333.

The Behavioral Health Education Center of Nebraska

A Creative Solution to a Persistent Behavioral Health Workforce Shortage

Emily Adams, MS[a], Shinobu Watanabe-Galloway, PhD[b],
Mogens Bill Baerentzen, PhD, CRC, LMHP[c], Allison Grennan, PhD[d],
Erin Obermeier Schneider, MSW[a], Marley Doyle, MD[a,*]

KEYWORDS

- Workforce development • Behavioral health • Continuing education

KEY POINTS

- States across the United States are faced with an inadequate supply of behavioral health professionals, especially in rural and urban underserved areas.
- Behavioral health professionals include psychiatrists, psychiatric physician assistants, psychiatric nurse practitioners, psychologists, mental health counselors, marriage and family therapists, clinical social workers, and substance use disorder counselors.
- The Behavioral Health Education Center of Nebraska (BHECN) was founded by the Nebraska legislature in 2009 to improve access to behavioral health care across the state by developing a skilled and passionate workforce.
- BHECN regularly reviews the changing characteristics of the behavioral health workforce, engages and recruits students to behavioral health majors, supports students completing training programs in behavioral health programs, and provides continuing education and support to retain practicing behavioral health professionals.

This article originally appeared in *Psychiatric Clinics*, Volume 45 Issue 2, June 2022.
[a] Behavioral Health Education Center of Nebraska, University of Nebraska Medical Center, 984242 Nebraska Medical Center, Omaha, NE 68198-4242, USA; [b] College of Public Health, University of Nebraska Medical Center, 984395 Nebraska Medical Center, Omaha, NE 68198, USA; [c] Mid-America Mental Health Technology Transfer Center, University of Nebraska Medical Center, 985450 Nebraska Medical Center, Omaha, NE 68198-5450, USA; [d] Munroe-Meyer Institute for Genetics and Rehabilitation, 985450 Nebraska Medical Center, Omaha, NE 68198-5450, USA
* Corresponding author.
E-mail address: marley.doyle@unmc.edu

INTRODUCTION

Behavioral health issues are highly prevalent in the United States. According to the latest national survey in 2019, approximately 51.5 million adults (20.6%, age 18 years and older) had any mental illness (AMI) in the United States, and an estimated 9.5 million adults (3.8%) had both AMI and at least one substance use disorder.[1–6] The United States has a widespread shortage of behavioral health providers, and people of color are less likely to have access to necessary services.[2] According to the Health Resources and Services Administration (HSRA) projections, by 2030, there may be a shortage of 14,300 psychologists, 34,940 addiction counselors, and 40,140 mental health counselors.[3,4,7]

Like many other rural states, Nebraska has faced a severe shortage of behavioral health providers. According to the most recently available data on the behavioral health workforce, 88 of Nebraska's 93 counties were designated as federal behavioral health professional shortage areas (HPSAs) in 2021.[6] Nebraska covers an area of 77,348 square miles, is home to 1.9 million people, and is mostly rural.[7] Of the 93 counties, 48 counties are classified as rural and 31 as frontier (having fewer than 7 residents per square mile).[8] Specifically, there is a behavioral workforce disparity within rural areas—for example, in rural Nebraska, there are only 2.7 psychiatrists per 100,000 residents compared with 11.3 psychiatrists per 100,000 residents in urban communities. Similar disparities are observed in other behavioral health professions such as psychologists (rural: 9.7 per 100,000; urban: 25.3 per 100,000) and licensed independent mental health practitioners (rural: 46.4 per 100,000; urban: 69.8 per 100,000).[9]

These behavioral health provider shortages are neither new to Nebraska nor unique compared to other states in the country. Although many states and communities have independently implemented efforts to attract and retain behavioral health workers, the success of these investments has varied and there remains no nationwide guidance on best practices for behavioral health workforce development. The current article will review the literature and present an in-depth review of one center's decade-long endeavor to strengthen the behavioral health workforce in Nebraska.

CURRENT STUDIES

The Annapolis Framework, a framework developed by the Substance Abuse and Mental Health Services Administration (SAMSHA) and the Annapolis Coalition, developed specific goals to address oral health workforce shortages, including broadening the concept of "workforce" (eg, including families, interprofessional collaboration); strengthening the workforce through federal, state, and local efforts; and creating structures to support the workforce (eg, establishing a financing system that adequately compensates the workforce). Workforce development, for the purposes of this article, is the attraction, development, and retention of behavioral health providers.

The behavioral health workforce shortage is more prevalent in rural communities than urban communities nationwide. It is estimated that 62% of mental HPSAs are in rural or partially rural areas.[10] Recruitment and retention of a competent rural behavioral health workforce is complicated by few financial incentives, perceived professional isolation, few academic behavioral health training programs in rural communities, limited access to continuous education and training, and limited exposure to the lifestyle in rural communities.[11–14] Likewise, there are not enough practitioners that specialize in specific populations (eg, geriatrics) and that represent the demographic diversity across the United States.[15] Specifically, people of color bear disproportionately high negative consequences stemming from a lack of access to behavioral health care and the subsequent downstream effects in other areas of life.[2]

A specific challenge to the behavioral health workforce is staff turnover. One study found rates of turnover among counselors at substance use disorder treatment programs as high as 74% over a 2-year period.[16] Another study reviewed existing literature on turnover in behavioral health fields and found 2 organization-level factors and 6 individual-level factors that contributed to turnover across studies.[17] Organizational culture and climate, the norms of a workplace, and employee perceptions of the workplace, respectively, were reported to impact the likelihood of turnover. Likewise, the individual factors that were found to contribute to turnover were stress/emotional exhaustion, a lack of organizational or social support, low job satisfaction, little job autonomy, limited or no growth opportunities, and the challenging nature of the work itself. Others echoed the findings that low job satisfaction contributed to turnover.[18] In addition, low approval of leadership, programs affiliated with a larger or parent organizations, and publicly owned programs were associated with greater turnover.

As part of a larger study on evidence-based practices (EBPs), quantitative and qualitative data were gathered regarding staff turnover at community-based behavioral health or child welfare agencies.[19] Employees younger in age and employees with lower job satisfaction were significantly more likely to turnover; having less than 1 year of tenure in the organization and having fewer years of tenure in the field overall were marginal predictors of turnover. The qualitative data gathered from individuals who left their agency indicated that job characteristics, such as the intense nature of the work and frequent evening, weekend, and on-call hours, contributed to their decision to leave the agency, as did low compensation, high requirements for productivity (ie, client-facing hours), a lack of advancement opportunities, and poor relationships with coworkers. Thus, the challenges to the behavioral health workforce seem to encompass individual, organizational, and occupational factors.

Recommendations from State-Specific Behavioral Health Workforce Investigations

Several states have conducted detailed analyses of behavioral health workforce shortages. Because there is no unified national approach to behavioral health workforce development, each effort reflects the unique challenges of the locale. Together, however, insights about more systematic challenges and opportunities to mitigate those challenges can be found.

In Washington State,[20] an assessment of the workforce resulted in recommendations that included a need for increased provider diversity, reimbursement and compensation commensurate to required education, and graduate school curriculum that reflects the changing landscape of modern mental health. These same recommendations were echoed by a similar study in California.[21] The cultural and linguistic competence of behavioral health practitioners is critical considering the diversity in the experience and expression of symptoms as well as the availability of diagnostic-supportive language to describe experiences.[2] For example, some American Indian and Alaska Native languages do not encompass words directly denoting depression and anxiety,[22] and African Americans are more often inaccurately diagnosed when presenting symptoms of depression.[23]

Nearby in Oregon,[24] an investigation found that solutions to addressing the behavioral health workforce shortage were better suited for managing certain aspects than others. For example, opportunities for professional development and career progression were successful incentives for retaining talent, whereas loan repayment was an attractive incentive to recruit providers but not to retain them. Likewise, Vermont's investigation[25] found licensure reciprocity, clinical internships with adequate supervision, and loan forgiveness to be effective recruitment tools. A virtual mentorship network in Nebraska links college and high school students with an interest in behavioral health careers with mentors. This program concluded that it is feasible to virtually connect mentors and rural students with an interest in behavioral health careers.[26] Virtual mentorship may be a promising avenue to encourage more people of color to become behavioral health practitioners, as people of color, and African Americans especially, tend to live in locations where fewer providers practice.[2]

Massachusetts, which has a relatively high density of psychiatrists, was home to a study[27] that pointed to structural challenges within and between agencies and insurance providers as a barrier to access care despite the adequate supply of providers. North Carolina's efforts[28] echoed others' calls for greater parity between job qualifications and compensation and highlighted the need for positive workplace cultures and greater access to clinical supervision.

New Mexico passed legislation in 2012 to systematically survey their behavioral health providers to better understand workforce shortages.[29] Survey findings indicated a shortage of providers representing diverse populations, limited services allowing for Medicaid and Medicare payors, a limited number of providers working in public health settings, and limited access to health information technology. Based on these findings, actions were grouped into 5 categories: a need for behavioral health workforce planning at the state level, a need to integrate primary care and behavioral health, a need to address the scarcity of independently licensed social workers and counselors in rural areas, a need to address shortages of behavioral health professionals through improved recruitment, and a need to improve behavioral health workforce retention. Innovative actions included: piloting telehealth supervision to rural clinicians, passage of a bill reducing barriers to licensure of applicants licensed in good standing in other jurisdictions, and passage of a bill making social workers and counselors eligible for rural practice state tax credits.

Programs that Address Behavioral Health Workforce Shortages

Several strategies to improve the rural behavioral health workforce shortage are described in the literature. An online behavioral health nurse practitioner program allows students to maintain employment and residence in rural communities while advancing their competencies to provide behavioral health care. Graduates from such programs might be more inclined to establish and maintain employment in a rural setting.[30] Financial assistance and loan forgiveness programs provide incentives for recent graduates to seek employment in rural and underserved communities, which is particularly helpful to increase recruitment of recent behavioral health graduates.[13,31]

Agencies in New York collaborated to identify ways social work graduates could be better prepared to implement EBPs upon entering the workforce.[32] Although EBPs are a gold standard in behavioral health, few are implemented with consistency and frequency, and it remains unclear how cultural factors influence the efficacy of EBPs.[2] The agencies engaged in strategic planning to develop a needs assessment, focus group, and survey to understand the perspectives of stakeholders at different points in the employee development process. Members of provider agencies and educational institutions provided input about skills being taught in training programs and skills needed in the workforce. This partnership between those who prepare students and those who hire students is a unique example of an opportunity to identify gaps in training that lead to solutions.[32]

In New Mexico, partnerships between stakeholders prepare third-year counseling psychology doctoral students for real-world situations in integrated health care teams.[33] A mix of intensive workshops and coursework help prepare students for working with nurses, physicians, and pharmacists with a focus on learning about the different professions and the unique perspectives each holds because of their training. This program prepares students for interprofessional collaboration and affords an opportunity for greater learning and respect for other professions, which can help reduce conflict and disagreements. Such integrated care facilities have the potential to bring greater benefit to people of color, as African Americans and Hispanic and Latino Americans are more likely to seek behavioral health care from a primary care provider than a specialist.[2,34] Likewise, New Mexico pioneered rural psychiatry residency rotations and recently found that residents who had completed a rural residency experience were more likely to practice in rural, frontier, or other underserved areas than residents who had not completed a rural residency.[35] Thus, the authors suggest that more psychiatry residents should have rural residency experiences to expose students to opportunities in areas of highest need.

The child and adolescent psychiatry telemental health program at the University of Hawaii built a model of serving rural sites and equipping those entering the workforce with experience in telehealth.[36] Their unique partnership with the local department of health, community health centers, and the Mayo Clinic offer psychiatry fellows an opportunity to engage with multidisciplinary teams to provide culturally competent care. A key element to the success of the program is having adequate resources to support the fellows in all aspects of their development and work. For example, treatment team meetings connect all professionals providing services to the child in a meeting that also includes their family. Likewise, clinical case consultation is available to fellows monthly through technology-assisted mediums, thereby reducing barriers to access for patients and fellows. This multidisciplinary approach focused on culturally competent care gives students a realistic preview of what serving in the rural community as a practitioner would entail.

BEHAVIORAL HEALTH EDUCATION CENTER OF NEBRASKA CONCEPTUAL MODEL

Although the previously reviewed literature offers insights into programs and studies that inform behavioral health workforce development efforts, few reports offered longitudinal evidence. One center in Nebraska has been operating for more than a decade to support the development of the behavioral health workforce in the state.

Nebraska reformed its state behavioral health system in 2004, and the Nebraska Legislature passed LB 1083,[37] which formally moved the state away from institutional care delivered at 3 state-run Regional Centers toward a community-based approach focused on maintaining wellness and recovery through resources in a person's home community. Despite Nebraska's progress in the last 10 years, a shortage of behavioral health professionals prevents people from getting the help they need when and where they need it.

To address this workforce shortage, the Nebraska Legislature passed LB 603 in 2009 and created the Behavioral Health Education Center of Nebraska (BHECN; Nebraska Revised Statute § 71–830).[38] BHECN's purpose is to recruit, retain, and increase competency of the state's licensed behavioral health workforce. To meet this purpose, BHECN collaborates with partners, listens to stakeholders, identifies resources and barriers, and includes consumers and families in their work. BHECN's goal is to provide accessible education and training to meet the needs of employers, behavioral health professionals, and consumers. They provide first-rate, interprofessional education services which satisfy the continuing education requirements for licensure and certification.

Fig. 1 shows the conceptual model that BHECN uses for programming and policy development. This conceptual model is based on the "leaky pipeline" model coined by researchers such as Pell[39] and Gasser[40] who studied the concern in lack of women in science, engineering, and technology careers. The model shows a linear progression through high school to full license acquisition and highlights how the individuals can be supported so that they will remain on the pathway to acquire the full license in behavioral health professions.

Behavioral Health Education Center of Nebraska Strategies and Outcomes

BHECN's mission is to improve access to behavioral health care across the state of Nebraska by developing a skilled and passionate workforce. To achieve this mission, BHECN identified 7 strategies and outcomes that guide their work, many of which are in progress or have been established.

1. *Behavioral health education and training sites in each region*: Develop 6 behavioral health regional sites to support local participation in interprofessional workforce development.
2. *Behavioral telehealth training*: Provide leadership and training in behavioral telehealth and other innovative means of care delivery to the entire behavioral health workforce.
3. *Interprofessional behavioral health training, curriculum development, and outcomes research*: Establish interprofessional collaborative partnerships to create, link, and disseminate education and training materials for the development of the behavioral health workforce, with emphasis on the recovery-focused needs of consumers.
4. *Fund psychiatry residents and other behavioral health trainees*: Fund additional psychiatric residents (2 each year, up to a total of 8) trained in interprofessional and telehealth service delivery to rural and underserved areas and facilitate funding of training for other behavioral health professions.

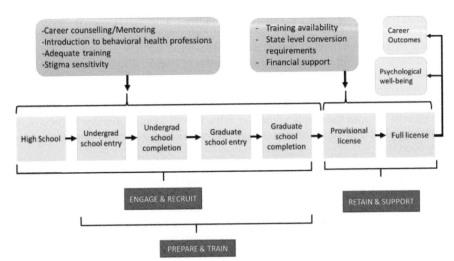

Fig. 1. Conceptual model that guides BHECN programming and policy development. Engagements occur at each of 3 levels: engage and recruit, prepare and train, and retain and support.

5. *Behavioral health workforce analysis*: Facilitate the collection, analysis, and dissemination of behavioral health workforce data and the prioritization of training and recruitment of behavioral health professionals by type and region.
6. *Networks*: Develop resource networks of highly committed, competent, and diverse individuals, committees, partners, and champions of behavioral health. The communication and education plan will foster access to resources to support and implement BHECN's mission and goals.
7. *Resources*: Build viable financial and operational infrastructure to meet the goals of BHECN's mission and fund its strategic initiatives.

Engage and Recruit

During the time from high school to undergraduate programs, it is necessary to actively engage with students in order to recruit them into pursuing a behavioral health career. Once they are in an undergraduate program and decide to pursue a behavioral health career, students should be supported to complete the program of study that is necessary for them to obtain an appropriate degree in behavioral health professions. Career counseling and mentorship play an important role in steering students into behavioral health professions. Behavioral health professionals may engage with students by giving a presentation or having a meeting with interested students to demystify behavioral health professions and reduce the stigma associated with behavioral health.

BHECN hosts a variety of presentations and conferences to introduce high school and college students to careers in behavioral health. BHECN's Ambassador Program was created in 2013 by former BHECN Director, Howard Liu, M.D., MBA, and BHECN Community Outreach Specialist, Ann Kraft, to introduce high school and college students to behavioral health careers and follow and support students through graduate and professional school. From 2010 to 2021, BHECN reached over 5000 high school and college students, including students from rural and urban underserved areas. BHECN also hosts yearly mentorship dinners, including interdisciplinary events to support students' networking with other students, behavioral health faculty, and practicing behavioral health professionals in the community. To complement their outreach efforts, BHECN created and distributed 10,000 copies of a brochure called Pathways to a Career in Behavioral Health, which details the education requirements, work environment, and projected growth of 8 different behavioral health careers (eg, psychiatrist, psychiatric nurse practitioner). In 2017 and 2018, BHECN funded community partners to engage youth in their area about careers in behavioral health.

Additional outreach to undergraduate and graduate students is achieved through the Nebraska Behavioral Health Education Partnership (NeBHEP), which was developed by BHECN's former Clinical Director, Joseph Evans, Ph.D., where BHECN and the 18 graduate-level behavioral health academic programs in the state collaborate to identify common programmatic challenges, challenges students face during and after their academic training, and solutions to better train the next generation of behavioral health care providers. A Psychiatry Interest Group helps keep regular communication with medical school students that have an interest in psychiatry with the goal of retaining psychiatrists in the state upon graduation. Students and professionals looking for new opportunities have access to NEBHjobs.com, a free resource for finding open jobs, and BHECN's Webinar Series: Core Topics for Behavioral Health Providers, which covers the latest developments in a range of essential behavioral health areas.

Prepare and Train

Upon completion of the degree program, the individual typically moves toward obtaining the provisional license (if needed). Depending on the profession, the time between the provisional license to full license can be anywhere between 2 and 5 years. Oftentimes, individuals have a difficult time finding a placement site and required supervision to earn necessary clinical hours; they may financially struggle because the positions available for a provisional license holder pay nothing or very low wages. As such, it is critical to provide necessary financial incentives and support as well as placement guidance to the individuals with provisional licenses.

As part of their training, up to 6 psychiatry residents have the opportunity to complete a BHECN-funded residency that includes opportunities to complete rotations in rural settings, giving residents a well-rounded experience and a chance to learn about the unique opportunities that exist in rural practice. Additional internship and training sites for behavioral health providers across a broad range of disciplines, including psychology, mental health counseling, addiction counseling, and physician assistant, expose students to rural and underserved communities. From 2017 to 2019, BHECN supported 132 students in graduate residency and internship training opportunities. BHECN also maintains strategic collaborations with interprofessional training sites and integrated behavioral health in primary care settings in both rural and urban areas to support students' development and comfort working in interprofessional settings.

Retain and Support

Even after the individual obtains the full license, supports are needed to retain the workforce; this is especially true with providers practicing in rural areas. BHECN works to engage with practicing behavioral health providers by providing continuing education and networking opportunities.

To support practicing behavioral health professionals, BHECN hosts or supports a diverse array of continuing education opportunities. In-person training opportunities have engaged subsets of the behavioral health workforce with didactic and professional development topics especially focused on discussing solutions to the workforce shortage in their field. Such topics have included learning opportunities on timely topics such as opioids, innovations in telehealth delivery, and self-care for professionals in behavioral health fields.

To reach a broader audience of practitioners across the state, BHECN offers many online trainings and webinars. Core Topics webinars support practitioners by delivering free educational material and continuing education credits on essential topics in behavioral health. In partnership with the Nebraska Department of Health and Human Services, Division of Behavioral Health and the University of Nebraska Medical Center (UNMC) Department of Psychiatry, BHECN established the Pain and Substance Use Disorder Project ECHO (Extension for Community Healthcare Outcomes); these webinars were attended by hundreds across the state.

In addition to the services that BHECN provides to students and practitioners, BHECN uses the Health Professions Tracking Service (HPTS) through the UNMC College of Public Health to track the behavioral health workforce distribution and licensure across Nebraska. The HPTS surveys licensed behavioral health practitioners from the Nebraska licensure database to learn about their work status, practice locations, and characteristics of the clients they see, which supplements the information that is collected through the licensure database. The resulting data set links personal and professional characteristics of the provider with details about the organizations they work for. Analyses of HPTS data have yielded insights that support BHECN's targeted recruitment and retention efforts. For example, 2018 analyses indicated that Nebraska's already limited behavioral health workforce is aging, with 58% of psychiatrists and 79% of LADCs above the age of 50 years.

A Decade of Progress

Through deliberate actions and coordinated collaboration, BHECN has enjoyed successes that have compounded over time, and BHECN is being recognized as a best practice in behavioral health workforce development, with other states modeling centers after it.[41,42] Since BHECN was founded in 2009 to address the state's shortage of behavioral health providers, Nebraska's behavioral health workforce has increased by 38%. More than 5200 students have participated in BHECN's Ambassador Program, increasing awareness of the opportunities that exist for students in behavioral health careers. Forty-three integrated behavioral health care in primary care clinics have been established in partnership with UNMC's Munroe-Meyer Institute, providing opportunities for hands on, interprofessional training opportunities across rural, underserved, and urban areas of the state. Of 41 behavioral health trainees who were placed in correctional and regional care center systems, 7 were hired for full-time positions. The NEBHjobs.com Web site has received more than 248,000 page views since it was created in 2015, connecting job seekers to opportunities in behavioral health fields. Recently, BHECN has expanded its partnership with academic training partners in the state to provide timely support to the immediate needs of students. Each year, BHECN celebrates the community by awarding students, community members, consumers, and distinguished professionals who have made a positive contribution to local behavioral health efforts. The accomplishments BHECN celebrates have been the result of intentional investment, cross-institutional collaboration, and dedicated teamwork. After more than a decade of dedicated effort, the successes of BHECN's efforts are being realized.

SUMMARY

The United States is currently experiencing a behavioral health access crisis in which the demand for behavioral health treatment is greater than the availability of behavioral health providers, especially in rural areas. BHECN can serve as a model for other states to implement similar programs to increase the availability of behavioral health care professionals and increase access to behavioral health services in their communities.

CLINICS CARE POINTS

- 62% of nationwide HPSAs are in rural or partially rural areas, and 88 of Nebraska's 93 counties were designated HPSAs in 2021.
- Often, the cultural and linguistic competency of behavioral health professionals does not match those seeking services.
- Students who have training experiences in rural areas may be more likely to establish and maintain employment in rural areas after graduation. Likewise, multidisciplinary training including telebehavioral health experiences are necessary building blocks for students.
- Partnerships across agencies are often necessary to provide necessary training opportunities for students.
- The Behavioral Health Education Center of Nebraska engages and recruits high school and undergraduate students to behavioral health programs, supports the preparation and training of behavioral health graduate students, and aids in retention and support of the existing behavioral health workforce.

DISCLOSURE

The authors have nothing to disclose.

REFERENCE

1. Substance Abuse and Mental Health Services Administration. Key substance use and mental health indicators in the United States: results from the 2019 national survey on drug use and health (HHS publication No. PEP20-07-01-001, NSDUH Series H-55). Rockville, MD: Center for Behavioral Health Statistics and Quality, Substance Abuse and Mental Health Services Administration; 2020. Available at: https://www.samhsa.gov/data/sites/default/files/reports/rpt29393/2019NSDUHFFRPDFWH TML/2019NSDUHFFR1PDFW090120.pdf. Accessed October 21, 2020.
2. Office of the Surgeon General (US); Center for Mental Health Services (US); National Institute of Mental Health (US). Mental health: culture, race, and ethnicity: a supplement to mental health: a report of the surgeon general. Rockville (MD): Substance Abuse and Mental Health Services Administration (US); 2001.
3. Health Resources and Services Administration. Behavioral Health Workforce Projections, 2016-2030: Clinical, Counseling, and School Psychologists. Available at: https://bhw.hrsa.gov/sites/default/files/bureau-health-workforce/data-research/psychologists-2018.pdf. Accessed October 21,2020.
4. Health Resources and Services Administration. Behavioral Health Workforce Projections, 2016-2030: Mental Health and School Counselors. Available at: https://bhw.hrsa.gov/sites/default/files/bureau-health-workforce/data-research/mental-health-and-school-counselors-2018.pdf. Accessed October 21,2020.
5. Health Resources & Services Administration. HPSA Find. Available at: https://data.hrsa.gov/tools/shortage-area/hpsa-find. Accessed September 1, 2021.
6. Dalstrom H, Naugle R. Britannica: Nebraska, state, United States. Available at: https://www.britannica.com/place/Nebraska-state. Accessed May, 14, 2020.
7. Health Resources and Services Administration. Behavioral Health Workforce Projections, 2016-2030: Addiction Counselors. Available at: https://bhw.hrsa.gov/sites/default/files/bureau-health-workforce/data-research/addiction-counselors-2018.pdf. Accessed October 21,2020.
8. Economic Research Service. Atlas of rural and small-town America. 2020. Available at: https://www.ers.usda.gov/data-products/atlas-of-rural-and-small-town-america/. Accessed May 1, 2020.
9. Behavioral Health Education Center of Nebraska. Workforce Reports. Available at: https://www.unmc.edu/bhecn/workforce/workforce-reports.html. Accessed October 20,2020.
10. Health Resources and Services Administration/Bureau of Health Workforce. Designated health professional shortage areas statistics: first quarter of fiscal year 2018 designated HPSA quarterly summary. Rockville, MD: HRSA; 2018. Available at: https://ersrs.hrsa.gov/ReportServer?/HGDW_Reports/BCD_HPSA/BCD_HPSA_SCR50_Qtr_Smry_HTML&rc:Toolbar=false. Accessed January 9, 2020.
11. Campbell N, McAllister L, Eley D. The influence of motivation in recruitment and retention of rural and remote allied health professionals: A literature review. Rural Remote Health 2012;12:1900.
12. Domino ME, Lin CC, Morrissey JP, et al. Training psychologists for rural practice: exploring opportunities and constraints. J Rural Health 2019;35(1):35–41.

13. Wantanabe-Galloway S, Madison L, Watkins KL, et al. Recruitment and retention of mental health care providers in rural Nebraska: perceptions of providers and administrators. Rural Remote Health 2015;15(4):3392.

14. Weinhold I, Gurtner S. Understanding shortages of sufficient health care in rural areas. Health Policy 2014;118(2):201–14.

15. Hoge MA, Stuart GW, Morris J, et al. Mental health and addiction workforce development: Federal leadership is needed to address the growing crisis. Health Aff 2013;32(11):2005–12.

16. Hatch-Maillette MA, Harwick R, Baer JS, et al. Counselor turnover in substance use disorder treatment research: Observations from one multisite trial. Subst Abus 2019;40(2):214–20.

17. Bernstein M. Shortage or maldistribution? Psychiatr Serv 2012;63(3):293.

18. Knight DK, Broome KM, Edwards JR, et al. Supervisory turnover in outpatient substance abuse treatment. J Behav Health Serv Res 2011;38(1):80–90.

19. Herschell AD, Kolko DJ, Hart JA, et al. Mixed method study of workforce turnover and evidence-based treatment implementation in community behavioral health care settings. Child Abuse Negl 2020;102.

20. Gattman NE, McCarty RL, Balassa A, et al. Washington state behavioral health workforce assessment. Olympia. WA: Washington Workforce Training and Education Coordinating Board; 2017. Available at: https://www.familymedicine.uw.edu/chws/wp-content/uploads/sites/5/2018/01/wa_bh_workforce_fr_dec_2017.pdf. Accessed March 26, 2021.

21. California Future Health Workforce Commission. Meeting the demand of health: final report of the California future health workforce commission 2019. Available at: https://futurehealthworkforce.org/our-work/final report/. Accessed March 26, 2021.

22. Manson SM. Ethnographic methods, cultural context, and mental illness: bridging different ways of knowing and experience. Ethos 1997;25:249–58.

23. Borowsky SJ, Rubenstein LV, Meredith LS, et al. Who is at risk of nondetection of mental health problems in primary care? J Gen Intern Med 2000;15:381–8.

24. Oregon Health Policy Board, Health Care Workforce Committee. Overview and recommendations for improving Oregon's provider incentive programs: report and recommendations for the Oregon Health Policy Board 2016. Available at: https://www.oregon.gov/oha/HPA/HP-HCW/Documents/Full%20OHPB%20File%20for%203396%20-%20PPT-Memo-Rept-App.pdf. Accessed April 12, 2021.

25. Vermont Department of Mental Health. Developmental disabilities and substance use disorder workforce report to Vermont legislature. 2017. Available at: https://legislature.vermo nt.gov/asset. Accessed April 12, 2021.

26. Keeler H, Sjuts T, Niitsu K, et al. Virtual mentorship network to address the rural shortage of mental health providers. Am J Prev Med 2018;54(6):290–5.

27. Citino C, Gibbons K, Hugo M, et al. The challenges of private practice: a study of clinicians' experiences providing mental health care in Massachusetts. Hadley MA: University of Massachusetts Donahue Institute; 2015. Available at: http://www.donahue.umassp.edu/documents/FINALCU_Report_4_21_15.pdf. Accessed April 19, 2021.

28. North Carolina Commission for Mental Health Developmental Disabilities and Substance Abuse Services. The joint workforce development initiative report 2008. Available at: https://www.ncleg.gov/documentsites/committees/JLOCMH-DD-SAS/LOC%20Minutes%20and%20Handouts/Minutes%20for%202008/April %2017,%202008/Workforce%20Development%20Plan-%20-S.%20Hairston %20-%20Attach.%20No.%204d.pdf. Accessed April 19, 2021.

29. Altschul DB, Bonham CA, Faulkner MJ, et al. State legislative approach to enumerating behavioral health workforce shortages: Lessons learned in New Mexico. Am J Prev Med 2018;54(6):220–9.
30. Sharp D, Bond M, Cheek K, et al. Quality of life impacts the recruitment and retention of rural health care providers. Natl Rural Health Assoc Policy Brief 2015;1–6.
31. Yanchus NJ, Periard D, Osatuke K. Further examination of predictors of turnover intention among mental health professionals. J Psychiatr Ment Health Nurs 2017; 24(1):41–56.
32. Easterly L. An educational model for workforce development: Dissemination of evidence-based practices. Community Ment Health J 2009;45:199–208.
33. Boland DH, Juntunen CL, Kim HY, et al. Integrated behavioral health curriculum in counseling psychology training programs. Couns Psychol 2019;47(7):1012–36.
34. Pingitore D, Snowden L, Sansone RA, et al. Persons with depressive symptoms and the treatments they receive: a comparison of primary care physicians and psychiatrists. Int J Psychiatry Med 2001;31(1):41–60.
35. Killough C, Ortegon ER, Vasireddy R, et al. Training psychiatrists in new mexico: reflections from psychiatry residents who participated in a rural track versus a traditional program alone over the past decade. Acad Psychiatry 2022;1–5. https://doi.org/10.1007/s40596-021-01572-2.
36. Alicata D, Schroepfer A, Unten T, et al. Telemental health training, team building, and workforce development in cultural context: The Hawaii experience. J Child Adolesc Psychopharmacol 2016;26(3):260–5.
37. Nebraska Legislative Bill 1083. Available at: https://nebraskalegislature.gov/FloorDocs/98/PDF/Slip/LB1083.pdf. Accessed April 19, 2021.
38. Nebraska Revised Statute 71-830. Available at: https://www.nebraskalegislature.gov/laws/statutes.php?statute=71-830. Accessed April 19, 2021.
39. Pell AN. Fixing the leaky pipeline: women scientists in academia. J Anim Sci 1996;74(11):2843–8.
40. Gasser CE, Shaffer KS. Career development of women in academia: Traversing the leaky pipeline. Prof Couns 2014;4(4):332–52.
41. Illinois Legislative Bill SB1979. Available at: https://www.ilga.gov/legislation/BillStatus.asp?DocNum=1979&GAID=16&DocTypeID=SB&LegId=134635&SessionID=110&GA=102. Accessed February 28, 2022.
42. Ormsby D. Senate OKs Fix to Illinois Behavioral Health Workforce Crisis. Patch.com. March 29. 2021. Available at: https://patch.com/illinois/springfield-il/senate-oks-fix-illinois-behavioral-health-workforce-crisis. Accessed February 28, 2022.

Gender Diversity in the Psychiatric Workforce
It's Still a (White) Man's World in Psychiatry

Crystal T. Clark, MD, MSc[a,b], Jennifer L. Payne, MD[c,*]

KEYWORDS

• Women • Psychiatry • BIPOC • Academia • United States • Inequity

KEY POINTS

- Although academic psychiatry has slightly higher rates of women at the Professor, Chair, and Endowed/Tenured Faculty ranks than academic medicine as a whole, women continue to be seriously underrepresented in upper ranks and leadership roles.
- Identified barriers include harassment and discrimination, gender bias in scholarly activities, Imposter Syndrome, lack of mentorship and sponsorship, work-life integration issues, and overinvolvement in nonpromotion academic activities.
- Psychiatry departments can take specific steps to level the playing field for women faculty to promote gender equity within their department.
- Reconstruction of Diversity, Equity, and Inclusion (DEI) roles will help advance recruitment and retention of women from BIPOC and other marginalized backgrounds.
- Gender equity is likely to lead to improved work-life balance and working conditions for both women and men as well as minorities.

INTRODUCTION: SCOPE OF THE PROBLEM

Since 2003, women and men have continued to apply to, enter, and graduate from medical school in similar proportions, and the percentage of full-time women faculty at US medical schools has gradually increased to a high of 43% in 2020.[1] Despite these advances, it is well known that women continue to be underrepresented in the highest academic rankings. Women make up the majority of the faculty at the Instructor level and, on par with their male counterparts, they represent approximately 50% of Assistant Professors. At the rank of Associate Professor, the percentage who

This article originally appeared in *Psychiatric Clinics*, Volume 45 Issue 2, June 2022.
 ᵃ Department of Psychiatry, University of Toronto, Women's College Hospital, 76 Grenville Street, Toronto, ON M5S 1B2, Canada; ᵇ Department of Obstetrics and Gynecology; ᶜ Department of Psychiatry and Neurobehavioral Sciences, University of Virginia, PO Box 800548, Charlottesville, VA 22908, USA
* Corresponding author.
E-mail addresses: crystal.clark@wchospital.ca (C.T.C.); Jlp4n@hscmail.mcc.virginia.edu (J.L.P.)

are women declines to 37%, and women only make up 25% of medical faculty who are Full Professors.[1] In academic medicine as a whole only 18% of all department chairs were held by women in 2018.[1]

Black, Indigenous and Persons of Color (BIPOC) who are women, specifically Black and Hispanic women, are underrepresented minorities in academic medicine. Black women represent 2.2% and Hispanic women make up 1.5% of all academic medical faculty. Similar to the trends in academic ranking of their White women counterparts, few are ranked Full Professor (Black 0.8%, Hispanic 1.0%) with a majority achieving the rank of Instructor (Black 3.0%, Hispanic 3.7%) and Assistant Professor (Black 3.2%, Hispanic 2.7%), and significantly fewer promoted to the rank of Associate Professor (Black 2.2%, Hispanic 1.5%). Only 0.7% of Black women are tenured compared with 19% of White women.[1]

But what about academic psychiatry—a field that might be considered kinder and gentler and perhaps a field that women might be drawn to? Sadly, academic psychiatry is only slightly better in gender equity than academic medicine. Although women make up 65% of Instructors in academic psychiatry, by the Professor level rank they are down to 37% and at the Chair level they make up 19.6%.[2] Similarly, in child and adolescent psychiatry, one of the most popular psychiatry subspecialties, 61% of trainees entering the field are women and they make up 58% of Lecturers, Instructors, and Assistant Professors as well as 53% of Associate Professors.[3] However, the percentage of women faculty sharply declines to 31% among Full Professors and 14% of Endowed Faculty.[3] Not unexpectedly, BIPOC women are inadequately represented compared with their White counterparts at every academic rank. Only 0.9% of psychiatry Professors are Black or Hispanic[1] and BIPOC women represent 6% of all chairs of psychiatry.[4]

The numbers in academic psychiatry are slightly better than academic medicine as a whole but they are still unacceptably low. Retention, advancement, and acknowledgment of the contributions of women faculty continue to be an obstacle. It is important that we, as a field, begin to examine the reasons for this inequity, the barriers to the advancement of women in academic psychiatry, and begin to build in solutions to correct this ongoing and self-perpetuating issue.

BARRIERS TO GENDER EQUITY

There are several different barriers that women face that put them at a disadvantage when it comes to academic advancement.

Harassment and Discrimination

Perhaps the most obvious and long-standing barrier is harassment and discrimination. There are several types of harassment and discrimination that women face: sexual harassment, gender-based discrimination, and maternal-based discrimination (defined as discrimination due to pregnancy, maternity leave, breastfeeding, or childcare issues). Although sexual harassment is frequently addressed in academic settings by trainings and clear policies and procedures for reporting, the other 2 types of discrimination are typically more subtle and can be even more psychologically damaging. Studies have found that 50% of women faculty and staff in academia have reported gender-based harassment by both superiors and peer faculty as well as by patients and others.[5] Another study found that two-thirds of physician mothers reported gender-based discrimination and one-third experienced maternal discrimination.[6] Although there are usually clear policies and procedures in place to report sexual harassment, gender and maternal discrimination often go unaddressed.

Studies have demonstrated that BIPOC women face more harassment than White women, White men, and BIPOC men because of the combined effects of sexual and racial discrimination.[7]

Gender Bias in Scholarship

Publications, citations, and funding awards are key metrics for achieving academic promotion. In 2018, women were 44.8% of first authors but, on trend with the disparity of women in senior leadership, only represented 35.7% of last authorships.[8] Even with near gender-parity for first authorships in psychiatry, data suggests that due to gender bias, articles authored by women are more likely to receive fewer citations.[8] In addition, women remain poorly represented on editorial boards, which impacts the type of publications accepted. Women researchers are less likely to be awarded NIH funding. Even when granted funding, women who are first-time principal investigators across all grant modalities on average are awarded significantly smaller grant amounts.[9] Research related to BIPOC mental health issues and health disparities and led by BIPOC faculty, especially Black and Hispanic women, have been less funded, which directly impacts promotion and tenure.[10] Similarly, publications on topics that BIPOC investigators more likely to research such as health disparities or community health research are less likely to be accepted for publication into high-impact journals.

Imposter Syndrome

Imposter Syndrome was first described in high achieving women[11] and refers to a pattern of behavior and thinking in which a person doubts their abilities and has fear of being exposed as an imposter or fraud despite evidence of success. Although this is an overgeneralization, it is thought that men tend to claim their success directly and women are more likely to discount their success by ascribing it to luck or to other factors. Imposter Syndrome is more common in women than in men. In a study of medical students, 50% of female students compared with 25% of male students were affected by Imposter Syndrome.[12] Imposter Syndrome leads to gender inequality in academia because it is associated with anxiety, depression, burnout, physical exhaustion, and avoidance of tasks with high prominence all of which deter promotion.[13,14]

Lack of Mentorship or Sponsorship

Mentorship and sponsorship are important keys to academic success. Mentorship is generally defined as a formal relationship for a period or for a particular project with a more senior or experienced person. Sponsorship, in contrast, is when a superior promotes a more junior person for various activities that can be helpful for the junior person's career—such as writing an article as a first author, presenting at a conference, or speaking at Grand Rounds. Male physicians are more likely to receive mentorship and sponsorship than female physicians and when women do have mentors or sponsors, they are less likely to be in powerful positions.[15–17] Compared with White women, Black women are less likely to receive sponsorship and struggle to find mentors from similar backgrounds because of a lack of BIPOC leadership representation. This "benign neglect" has a direct effect on impairing promotion of women both in terms of rank and into leadership roles.

Work-Life Integration Issues

Although there have been advances in maternity and family leave policies, policies remain inconsistent across academia.[17] Despite greater representation of women in the workforce, childcare responsibilities still often fall primarily on women and the childbearing years for women generally occur right at the peak of when young academics need to concentrate on building their careers. These inequities contribute to the slower pace of women's careers in academic medicine. In addition, BIPOC women physicians serve disproportionately as caregivers to parents and extended family. First-generation BIPOC women physicians may also carry the burden of more student loans and financially aiding extended family members, which results in additional burden and focus on activities that maximize compensation. These burdens are compounded by gender pay gaps and the added responsibilities are not factored into productivity nor have there been concerted efforts to reduce burnout in this particular population of physicians.

Overinvolvement in Nonpromotion Activities

At least partially due to a lack of mentorship, women often participate in activities that are necessary within a department but that are not valued for promotion. Women disproportionately contribute more time to clinical care, teaching, and service for academic medical centers.[18] Although these activities are vital to the institution/department missions and operations, they are not valued in the same way as research activities for advancement. Although most academic psychiatrists see patients, seeing more patients takes time away from activities that do promote advancements such as writing articles and grants. Educational contributions such as curriculum development, lecturing, and supervising medical students, residents, and fellows are time-consuming. Other activities such as serving on committees can be distractions as well. Although all inexperienced faculty are susceptible to this problem, women, particularly in the setting of inadequate mentorship, can be particularly vulnerable. BIPOC women are more likely to be requested to commit to uncompensated obligations that are completed outside of their main roles and in some cases, outside of their academic expertise, including development of curriculum that addresses health disparities, lecturing or providing perspective on antiracism efforts, serving as the "diverse" faculty member on departmental/institution committees, and supervision of trainees. These are all activities that are not valued for promotion. This "minority tax" undermines BIPOC women's abilities to focus on promotion-generating activities.

SOLUTIONS FOR THE ADVANCEMENT OF WOMEN

There are several approaches that psychiatry departments can take to eliminate gender disparities and to promote the careers of women and BIPOC women.

Eliminate Gender Pay Gap

Eliminating the gender pay gap by developing transparent salary and promotion processes ultimately helps everyone in academia, regardless of gender. However, equalizing compensation between the sexes will give women in academia more financial freedom to say no to activities that are not helpful toward promotion and to smooth out work-life integration. Being able to afford help at home whether in childcare, elderly care, cleaning, or other household duties can give a young academic the ability to concentrate on activities that are important for building her career.

Address Harassment and Implicit Bias

Institutions can address harassment and implicit bias against women in numerous ways. These practices generally improve the environment for everyone including men and women as well as BIPOC and those with other marginalized identities (eg, sexual orientation, religion, disability). Training that directly addresses harassment and implicit bias is a critical component of reducing harassment and bias. Most academic institutions administer antibias and antiharassment learning modules digitally. These serve as "check the box" efforts to reduce harassment and bias but fall short of the important group dialogue necessary to strengthen learning and foster the self-reflection essential for changes in thinking and behavior. Training mandates for all levels of leadership and faculty and frequent review are imperative. In addition, assessment of outcomes including external feedback is crucial to determine whether harassment and bias experiences are reduced and to evaluate achievement of institutional and departmental antibias and antiharassment goals. Implementation of other policies that truly address these issues is crucial. These include "open door and zero tolerance" policies, promoting a culture where individuals feel they can speak up about harassment and empowering the community with the responsibility to reduce, prevent, and report sexual harassment. Diversity, equity, and inclusion (DEI) committees, offices, or individuals charged with addressing these issues can serve the purpose of addressing issues of harassment and discrimination at an institutional level and bring these issues into focus on a regular basis.

Develop "Male Allies" Within the Department

In addition to working toward eliminating harassment and implicit bias, departments can advocate for, from a more positive perspective, male allies within the department who use deliberate action to promote gender equity.[19] These men leverage power and influence to make sure that women are "at the table" for major decisions, leadership opportunities, awards, and speaking engagements. They also credit women for their work and ideas and are intentional in advocating for women colleagues.

Leadership Training for Women

One approach to eliminating barriers for women in academia is to provide leadership training specifically for women. These programs can help address inadequate mentorship and level the playing field for women by providing practical advice, insight into individual strengths and weaknesses, and development of specific skills for leadership. Ideally, leadership training for women should take place at all rank levels as women at different levels of rank will have different needs to be addressed. Leadership training should be linked with identified career development goals at each rank. These programs are one way of addressing Imposter Syndrome and, in addition, leadership programs provide opportunities for women to meet other women in similar circumstances, which can provide a sense of community, resources of support, and idea-sharing for common problems.

Mentorship Programs

Mentorship is not necessarily intuitive. Being a good mentor, and just as important, a good mentee, are skills that can be taught. Having mentorship training, and requiring faculty members to take it, are other ways that academic departments can address gender inequity. It is also important to develop formal mentorship programs with opportunities for women to have access to mentors in more powerful positions. When departments prioritize mentorship and ideally financially support time for mentorship activities, everyone benefits.

Add Gender Equalizing Processes to Promotions/Awards

Another technique that academic departments can use to minimize barriers for women is to add gender equalizing processes to the promotion process, awards, and other application processes. For example, making sure that positions are advertised to all faculty members in a department and not just to a select few, having a formal application process for positions and awards, and preferably having a diverse committee to decide the outcomes of position and award applications can make these processes fairer for everyone. Including a "stop the clock" policy for promotion when young faculty members of either sex have children is another technique. Awards committees can include in their deliberations time taken off for family leave when judging how productive a candidate has been. These approaches can help academic departments improve inclusion not just for women but members of other minority populations as well.

Redefining What Contributions Are Valued for Promotion

Clinical and educational roles, disproportionately served by women and BIPOC, have historically been undervalued. These vital components of academic institutions deserve more recognition. Clinician-educators are increasingly burned out by clinical care demands and uncompensated educational obligations, which results in less retention of these faculty members. Furthermore, formal mentorship for writing and publishing in education is generally less available for clinician-educators. Compensation, allotted time, and well-defined promotion metrics to achieve full professorship for contributions to education including teaching and supervising trainees would help to reduce inequalities in academic rank for women and BIPOC who prefer to serve as clinician-educators.

Diversity, Equity, and Inclusion Reconstruction

DEI roles in medical institutions were developed to support policies and programs that address inequities among diverse identities (ie, gender, race/ethnicity, sexual orientation, religion, age, disability). However, these roles have often been tokenized and frequently lack the power structure, financial support, administrative resources, and protected time to be most effective. A recent guideline by national DEI leaders recommends that to increase diversity in leadership by women, including those who are BIPOC and LGBTQ+, a reconstruction of the DEI position for many departments is required.[20] These advised best practices to effectively support DEI leadership efforts include:

- Recognition of the role: Recognition can include changes in title, making the DEI role part of the departmental leadership team, and awarding of endowed chairs for the DEI role. These practices will help demonstrate departmental commitment and will elevate visibility and academic prestige of the DEI role.
- Allocation of financial support and resources: Financial salary support will provide protected time and clear institutional commitment for the role. Just as important, dedicated discretionary funding as well as administrative staff for regular and strategic programming and services will allow DEI leaders to make real differences in DEI issues that impact the department and medical institutions at large.
- Clearly defined duties of the role: By clearly defining duties of the DEI role and providing commiserate salary support, the DEI leader will be empowered to make the necessary changes directly tied to defined goals for the department. Other recommendations include a reporting structure to include the Department Chair and the Dean of the school, creating a Diversity Committee to support the DEI leader, a selection process on par with the department process for vice-chairs, professional development and leadership skills training, and term limits and evaluation at clearly defined points.

These practices will protect and support the DEI leader, moving them from a token position to a position of power and leadership to effect change within the department.

SUMMARY

Although academic psychiatry is marginally better than academic medicine as whole, women and BIPOC women continue to be underrepresented in the higher ranks and leadership positions in academic psychiatry departments. There are numerous barriers that influence the lack of career progression for women ranging from harassment and discrimination, lack of mentorship, life integration issues, and participation in non–promotion-generating academic activities that slow women's career progression. In addition, Impostor Syndrome is more common in women, which also hinders a woman's confidence in her abilities to generate promotion-supporting activities. The slower rate of promotion of women to higher ranks results in a vicious cycle of a lack of successful senior women who can in turn mentor younger women. A thoughtful approach to increasing both gender and minority diversity at upper ranks and in leadership is needed and will improve the academic culture across the board for everyone, including men. Similar to the need to reconstruct the DEI role in departments in order to support the role in achieving the goals of DEI, redesigning academia to not just value research but to also value education and clinical care will improve the academic environment for all academic psychiatrists. Providing the resources to support those in education, clinical care, and providing mentorship to others will increase the likelihood that women are not only promoted faster and have more successful careers, but will also be able to provide mentorship to others and to add their voices to leadership roles. It is our hope that academic psychiatry will become a model for other academic departments in how to support women and BIPOC women to have successful academic careers and to promote their leadership within departments and medical schools. It is time for psychiatry departments to take a serious look at what has been the traditional approach to academia and to redesign their processes, resource allocation, and overemphasis on research for promotion to promote diversity in leadership.

DISCLOSURE

The authors have nothing to disclose.

REFERENCES

1. AAMC. Faculty roster. 2019. U.S. Medical School Faculty. https://www.aamc.org/data-reports/faculty-institutions/interactive-data/2019-us-medical-school-faculty?msclkid=690bd108b67011ec9873ced53e27472
2. Chaudhary AMD, Naveed S, Siddiqi J, et al. US psychiatry faculty: academic rank, gender and racial profile. Acad Psychiatry 2020;44(3):260–6.
3. Hosoda M, Veenstra-VanderWeele J, Stroeh OM. Gender disparities in the child psychiatry ranks. J Am Acad Child Adolesc Psychiatry 2021;60(7):793–5.
4. Borlik MF, Godoy SM, Wadell PM, et al. Women in academic psychiatry: inequities, barriers, and promising solutions. Acad Psychiatry 2021;45(1):110–9.
5. Golden SH. The perils of intersectionality: racial and sexual harassment in medicine. J Clin Invest 2019;129(9):3465–7.
6. Adesoye T, Mangurian C, Choo EK, et al. Perceived discrimination experienced by physician mothers and desired workplace changes: a cross-sectional survey. JAMA Intern Med 2017;177(7):1033–6.

7. National Academies of Sciences, Engineering, and Medicine; Policy and Global Affairs; Committee on Women in Science, Engineering, and Medicine; Committee on the Impacts of Sexual Harassment in Academia. In: Benya FF, Widnall SE, Johnson PA, editors. Sexual Harassment of Women: Climate, Culture, and Consequences in Academic Sciences, Engineering, and Medicine. Washington (DC): National Academies Press (US) Copyright by the National Academy of Sciences. All Rights Reserved; 2018.

8. Hart KL, Frangou S, Perlis RH. Gender trends in authorship in psychiatry journals from 2008 to 2018. Biol Psychiatry 2019;86(8):639–46.

9. Oliveira DFM, Ma Y, Woodruff TK, et al. Comparison of national institutes of health grant amounts to first-time male and female principal investigators. JAMA 2019; 321(9):898–900.

10. Hoppe TA, Litovitz A, Willis KA, et al. Topic choice contributes to the lower rate of NIH awards to African-American/black scientists. Sci Adv 2019;5(10):eaaw7238. https://doi.org/10.1126/sciadv.aaw7238.

11. Clance PR, Imes SA. The imposter phenomenon in high achieving women: dynamics and therapeutic intervention. Psychotherapy 1978;15:241–7.

12. Villwock JA, Sobin LB, Koester LA, et al. Impostor syndrome and burnout among American medical students: a pilot study. Int J Med Educ 2016;7:364–9.

13. Seritan AL, Mehta MM. Thorny Laurels: the Impostor Phenomenon in Academic Psychiatry. Acad Psychiatry 2016;40(3):418–21.

14. Bravata DM, Watts SA, Keefer AL, et al. Prevalence, predictors, and treatment of impostor syndrome: a systematic review. J Gen Intern Med 2020;35(4):1252–75.

15. Carr PL, Gunn C, Raj A, et al. Recruitment, promotion, and retention of women in academic medicine: how institutions are addressing gender disparities. Womens Health Issues 2017;27(3):374–81.

16. Farkas AH, Bonifacino E, Turner R, et al. Mentorship of women in academic medicine: a systematic review. J Gen Intern Med 2019;34(7):1322–9.

17. Riano NS, Linos E, Accurso EC, et al. Paid family and childbearing leave policies at top US medical schools. JAMA 2018;319(6):611–4.

18. Jena AB, Khullar D, Ho O, et al. Sex differences in academic rank in US medical schools in 2014. JAMA 2015;314(11):1149–58.

19. Jain S, Madani K, Flint L, et al. What does it mean to be a male ally? Implementing meaningful change in gender representation in medicine. J Am Coll Surg 2020; 230(3):355–6.

20. Jordan A, Shim RS, Rodriguez CI, et al. Psychiatry diversity leadership in academic medicine: guidelines for success. Am J Psychiatry 2021;178(3):224–8.

Disability Inclusion in Psychiatry

Strategies to Improve and Increase Diversity Within the Psychiatrist Workforce

Marley Doyle, MD

KEYWORDS

- Psychiatry • Disability • Inclusion • Diversity

KEY POINTS

- The number of Psychiatry residents and Psychiatrists with disabilities is not well studied.
- Mental health providers with disabilities can add value to medical student and resident education.
- The inclusion of mental health providers with disabilities can improve the quality of patient care.

VIGNETTE

I am a blind psychiatrist and have struggled with integrating my identity as a physician and a person with a disability throughout my medical training and practice—these identities are not often married in the minds of medicine.

As a fellow, I was preparing for a new patient evaluation in the outpatient clinic. My patient, a 21-year-old woman with a history of major depressive disorder (MDD) and generalized anxiety disorder (GAD), presented with worsening depressive symptoms in the context of academic difficulties. During the evaluation, I learned that this patient, a person with a visual disability, was having difficulty securing accommodations at her university. She felt frustrated, expressing her feelings of being marginalized she said, "*I guess I just don't belong and don't know why I try.*" As a physician living with blindness, I could relate to this patient. We made a treatment plan and agreed to a follow-up appointment in 2 weeks. As she was leaving the appointment, she looked at my computer screen and said, "*You use a screen reader? I knew there was a reason you understood me!*". As our relationship evolved, I became more comfortable

This article originally appeared in *Psychiatric Clinics*, Volume 45 Issue 2, June 2022.
University of Nebraska Medical Center, 985575 Nebraska Medical Center, Omaha, NE 68798, USA
E-mail address: Marley.Doyle@unmc.edu

Child Adolesc Psychiatric Clin N Am 33 (2024) 53–56
https://doi.org/10.1016/j.chc.2023.06.006
1056-4993/24/© 2023 Elsevier Inc. All rights reserved.

disclosing my visual impairment and sharing strategies that I had found helpful. In retrospect, the most therapeutic piece of our work together was the patient's ability to receive care from a medical professional with a disability. I believe this allowed her to visualize herself as a capable student who could plan a future that included multiple career options. The patient's grades improved through the year, and she was able to enroll in her final semester of college. I think about this patient often, as I reflect on how a chance encounter led to mutual benefit. I was able to offer her hope that as a person with a disability, she was able to aspire to advanced education, and my patient allowed me to change my perspective. My disability could be a potential strength, rather than something that needed to remain hidden. This was the first time I realized that my disability could benefit my patients because I could offer them a unique vantage point and approach rooted in a deep understanding of disability—unfortunately, the pathway to medicine lacks physicians with disabilities. Why are these physicians important and how can we increase the inclusion of this valuable and diverse group?

WHY ARE PHYSICIANS WITH DISABILITIES IMPORTANT?
Informed Care

The current health-care system is not well equipped to assess and treat the needs of patients with disabilities. Although chronic illness and disability are sequelae of many medical illnesses, the response has been sluggish with little to no attention paid to ensuring easy access to care. As mentioned above, I am a physician with blindness, which also means that I am a patient. At each ophthalmology appointment, I am invariably handed paper forms to fill out, and I am met with surprise when I inform them that I cannot read the paperwork. I have never been asked whether I need accommodations before an appointment and am frequently frustrated and dismayed by the lack of knowledge of health-care providers when it comes to understanding my disability. I can only imagine the frustration and disempowerment felt by a patient who does not have a medical background and is expected to navigate the system. The mental health-care system is notoriously difficult to navigate with numerous barriers to care. This becomes even more trying for patients who have psychiatric disabilities who are often met with long wait-times and a complicated referral process. The health-care system, including mental health-care, is reaching a critical tipping point—an imminent need for more psychiatrists and the need to provide more diverse and informed care in the workforce. This tipping point is a keen opportunity to reframe historical perceptions of diversity and to intentionally, and strategically, grow the diversity of psychiatrists—especially those with disability.

INCREASE IN MENTAL HEALTH NEEDS AND DECLINE IN PSYCHIATRISTS

In 2019, 51.5 million adults aged 18 years or older in the United States were estimated to have a mental illness. This represents 20.6% of all US adults. In the past year, less than half (44.8%) of these adults received mental health services.[1] This means that there are nearly 23 million Americans with a mental illness who are not receiving any treatment. In 2019, 61 million (26%) US adults were reported having a disability, including mental health disabilities.[2] Persons with disabilities are more likely to experience mental health conditions, so psychiatrists need to be well versed in the treatment of patients with both psychiatric disorders and disability. In addition, psychiatrists with disabilities should be adequately represented in the workforce to assure their perspectives are represented.

The workforce needs for psychiatrists will soon be exceedingly unmet. The Health Resources and Services Administration estimated a total of 33,650 adult psychiatrists and 8090 child and adolescent psychiatrists in 2020. By 2030, a 20% decrease is predicted in adult psychiatrists; 22% in child and adolescent providers. Concurrent to these decreases is a 3% increase in demand for mental health services.[3]

BUILDING AN INCLUSIVE WORKFORCE

Psychiatry is tasked with implementing strategic, inclusive workforce development strategies to meet the needs of the population. To meet this goal, recruitment efforts will need to focus on increasing the number of medical students interested in psychiatry but will also need to examine the demographic characteristics of these students to ensure that the workforce adequately represents the population treated. In the past decade, there has been a burgeoning focus on diversity within the medical field, and now is the time to include people with disabilities in the discussion.

The number of medical professionals with disabilities has only recently been reported. According to an anonymous survey, 7.6% of graduating medical students, and 3.1% of attending physicians disclose disability.[4,5] A dearth of data exists on the status of disability among residents with only one survey of Emergency Medicine residents in which 4.1% disclosed a disability.[6] To our knowledge, no data exists on the number of psychiatrists with disabilities.

A concerning trend emerges showing a decrease with fewer attending physicians reporting a disability compared with medical students. Although the exact cause for the decline is uncertain, we suspect several contributing factors including lack of mentorship, lack of support within the medical education and health-care systems, and lack of targeted strategies to specifically include those with disabilities.

Although the American Psychiatric Association currently supports a Workforce Inclusion Pipeline Program and caucuses for underrepresented racial and ethnic minorities, no such programs exist for students or psychiatrists with disabilities.[7–9] Student engagement is an important part of workforce development but we also recognize that recruitment into the psychiatric workforce is not ideal if there are few mentors that have disabilities. Attention to current psychiatrists with disabilities is also of utmost importance and can be accomplished by accommodation support and peer mentorship. In recent years, social media campaigns such as #DocsWithDisabilties and #FutureDocsWithDisabilities have increased awareness of the presence of medical students and physicians with disabilities, as well as promoting advocacy within medical education and practice. In addition, those in leadership must also ensure the inclusion of those with disabilities to help ensure that decisions made consider diverse perspectives. Finally, medical student education must address disability for providers without disabilities to better understand and treat patients with disabilities.

SUMMARY

Although there is much work to be done, we believe that inclusion needs to begin at some point and want to advocate that psychiatrists with disabilities are included in diversity, equity, and inclusion efforts across the field. In the context of the current and projected psychiatric shortage, it is of utmost importance that we include people from all backgrounds to enhance the experience of psychiatrists and patients alike.

Consider adding to conclusion a comment on whether there is a need for a comprehensive curriculum on disability for medical educators, program directors, and psychiatric leaders.

CLINICS CARE POINTS

- Don't assume everyone is able-bodied. Be upfront about need for accommodations.
- Include peole with disabilities on Diversity, Equity and Inclusion Committees.

DISCLOSURE

The author has no commercial or financial conflicts of interest or any funding sources.

REFERENCES

1. Substance Abuse and Mental Health Services Administration. Key substance use and mental health indicators in the United States: Results from the 2019 National survey on Drug Use and health (HHS Publication No. PEP20-07-01-001). Rockville, MD: Center for Behavioral Health Statistics and Quality; 2020. Substance Abuse and Mental Health Services Administration. Available at: https://www.samhsa.gov/data/sites/default/files/reports/rpt29393/2019NSDUHFFRPDFWHTML/2019NSDUHFFR1PDFW090120.pdf.
2. Okoro CA, Hollis ND, Cyrus AC, et al. Prevalence of Disabilities and Health Care Access by Disability Status and Type Among Adults — United States, 2016. MMWR Morb Mortal Wkly Rep 2018;67:882–7. https://doi.org/10.15585/mmwr.mm6732a3.
3. U.S. Department of Health and Human Services, Health Resources and Services Administration, National Center for Health Workforce Analysis, National Projections of Supply and Demand for Selected Behavioral Health Practitioners: 2013-2025. Available at: https://bhw.hrsa.gov/sites/default/files/bhw/health-workforce-analysis/research/projections/behavioral-health2013-2025.pdf.
4. Meeks LM, Case B, Plegue M, et al. National Prevalence of Disability and Clinical Accommodations in Medical Education. J Med Educ Curric Dev 2020;7. https://doi.org/10.1177/2382120520965249. 2382120520965249.
5. Nouri Z, Dill MJ, Conrad SS, et al. Estimated Prevalence of US Physicians With Disabilities. JAMA Netw Open 2021;4(3):e211254. https://doi.org/10.1001/jamanetworkopen.2021.1254.
6. Sapp RW, Sebok-Syer SS, Gisondi MA, et al. The Prevalence of Disability Health Training and Residents With Disabilities in Emergency Medicine Residency Programs. AEM Educ Train 2020;5(2):e10511.
7. Saha S, Komaromy M, Koepsell TD, et al. Patient-physician racial concordance and the perceived quality and use of health care. Arch Intern Med 1999;159(9):997–1004.
8. American Psychiatric Association. Workforce Inclusion Pipeline Programs. 2021. Available at: https://www.psychiatry.org/residents-medical-students/medical-students/medical-student-programs/workforce-inclusion-pipeline.
9. Swenor B, Meeks LM. Disability Inclusion - Moving Beyond Mission Statements. N Engl J Med 2019;380(22):2089–91.

Building a Diverse Psychiatric Workforce for the Future and Helping Them Thrive

Recommendations for Psychiatry Training Directors

Asale Hubbard, PhD[a,b,1], Andrew Sudler, MD, MPH[a],
Jean-Marie E. Alves-Bradford, MD[c], Nhi-Ha Trinh, MD, MPH[d,2],
Anne D. Emmerich, MD[d,3], Christina Mangurian, MD, MAS[a,*]

KEYWORDS

- Workforce diversity • Psychiatry residency training
- Psychiatry residency recruitment • Training directors • Anti-racism
- Structural competency

KEY POINTS

- The development of intentional recruitment pipelines at universities, outreach to minority-serving universities, and examination of selection strategies to reduce bias are essential to increasing underrepresented in medicine (URM) enrollment in psychiatry training programs.
- Retention of URM trainees is strengthened through the creation of affinity group spaces, structured opportunities, and mentorship with URM faculty and consideration of policies and/or potential barriers to the success of URM trainees.
- Training programs must move beyond cultural factors to examine how structural forces impact the experience of health care. Training curriculums should include a focus on structural competency, provide opportunities to engage in advocacy, and the development of research centered on participation of the communities of interest.

This article originally appeared in *Psychiatric Clinics*, Volume 45 Issue 2, June 2022.
^a University of California, San Francisco Department of Psychiatry and Behavioral Sciences, Weill Institute for Neurosciences, 675 18th Street, San Francisco, CA 94107, USA; ^b San Francisco VA Health Care System; ^c Columbia University Department of Psychiatry, 1051 Riverside Drive Box 112, New York, NY 10032, USA; ^d Massachusetts General Hospital Department of Psychiatry
¹ Present address: 4150 Clement Street (116B), San Francisco, CA 94121.
² Present address: One Bowdoin Square, Boston, MA 02114.
³ Present address: 15 Parkman Street, Boston, MA 02114.
* Corresponding author.
E-mail address: christina.mangurian@ucsf.edu
Twitter: @cmangurian (C.M.)

Child Adolesc Psychiatric Clin N Am 33 (2024) 57–69
https://doi.org/10.1016/j.chc.2023.06.007
1056-4993/24/© 2023 Elsevier Inc. All rights reserved.

childpsych.theclinics.com

INTRODUCTION

In 2020, our world irrevocably changed because of the COVID-19 pandemic. Concurrently, in the United States, racial uprisings following the murder of Mr George Floyd and the losses of other innocent Black lives cast a spotlight on the syndemic of COVID-19 and structural racism. This spotlight has galvanized health care institutions to re-examine and renew their commitment to Diversity, Equity, and Inclusion (DEI) with a sharper focus on antiracism efforts.

Demographic shifts in our population over the past few decades also argue for this. Per 2020 census data, only 60% of Americans now identify as White, compared with 80% in 1980.[1] The Pew Center reports that 46.8 million Americans (14% of the population) identified as Black in 2019, an increase of 29% since 2000.[2] More than 50% of young people under the age of 16 years now identify as belonging to one or more racial or ethnic minority groups.[1] Census data estimates predict that by 2043, non-White people will make up more than one-half of the overall US population.[3] A report by Wilson estimates that the shift to a non-White majority working class (defined as people without a college degree, who make up two-third of the workforce) will occur much earlier, in 2032, only 11 years from now.[3]

Despite the shifting demographics in the United States, many Black, Indigenous, People of Color (BIPOC) communities remain marginalized and significant inequities exist in medical and mental health care. Increasing evidence shows that implicit bias by majority clinicians is one of the many reasons why health inequities exist in communities of color.[4] Patients are increasingly requesting access to clinicians from BIPOC communities, and studies support the concept that this can contribute to better treatment outcomes.[5,6] Population demographics are shifting toward a non-White majority, but the demographics of psychiatrists and psychologists are not. We face a diversity crisis in mental health professions. Per an American Psychiatric Association report, the number of psychiatry trainees overall in the United States increased by 20.7% between 2014 and 2018 (to 6247),[7] but *"the racial and ethnic diversity among psychiatric trainees has not changed significantly since 2016."*[8]

In 2018, fewer than 10% of incoming PGY-1 psychiatry residents self-identified as Black/African American and Hispanic/Latino/Spanish Origin. Less than 1% self-identified as American Indian/Alaskan Native or Native Hawaiian/Other Pacific Islander.[8] In 2018, only 7% of US psychiatrists were Black.[9]

Even if the number of BIPOC individuals entering mental health professional training programs increases, it will still take years for the overall availability of licensed BIPOC clinicians in the community to change and training programs are the only mechanism through which this need can be addressed. Lin, Stamm, and Christidis report that although one-third of psychology PhDs were awarded to students who identified as racial/ethnic minorities in 2016, the overall percentage of White psychologists in practice remained 86%.[10] The average medical school graduate takes 4 to 6 years or more to complete psychiatric residency and subspecialty fellowship training and both during and after training, there are geographic inequities in the availability of underrepresented minority (URM) clinicians. A 2019 Association of Medical Colleges Report on Residents shows that 64.5% of psychiatry residents remain in the state in which they trained after completion of residency and across specialties women are more likely to remain in the state in which they trained.[11]

Trainees are not uniformly represented in all parts of the country and psychiatrists, in general, are often scarce in parts of the country with the most significant percentages of non-White residents. The American Psychiatric Association 2019 Resident/Fellow Census[8] stated: *"There are large differences across states in the number of psychiatry trainees per capita. The District of Columbia, New York, and Massachusetts have the largest number of per capita trainees. At the same time, parts of the southern and western U.S. tend to have insufficient numbers of per capita trainees."* Some states, including Arkansas, Idaho, Montana, and Wyoming had no new trainees enter psychiatry training programs in 2018.[8]

In addition, significant challenges exist for psychiatric training programs attempting to recruit BIPOC candidates. The most challenging is gaps in the pipeline. We must find ways to give young people exposure to STEM careers—particularly mental health—in elementary and high school, supporting them to keep alive their dream of going to medical school throughout college, and providing outstanding mentorship, nurturance, support in medical school, and residency, fellowship, and later.

For the 5% of medical school graduates who do choose to enter psychiatry each year,[7] considerations such as the lower expected income for psychiatrists compared with other specialties can be a barrier. This is a major problem diversifying our field, given that Black medical students owe more on average than students from other groups. Estimates indicate that over 50% of Black medical students graduate with more than $200,000 in debt, and 17% graduate with over $300,000 in debt.[12]

Once recruited, programs also face challenges with retaining trainees who have often become discouraged by bias and microaggressions during the training years.[13] Many BIPOC psychiatrists are also without culturally congruent mentorship. They are vulnerable to being asked to take on more than their share of diversity-related work by their institution, usually with little compensation (often called the minority tax).[14] In addition, given the small numbers of BIPOC trainees, the experience of imposter syndrome is common, again leading to difficulty with later faculty retention and feeling of thriving. In fact, Jordan and colleagues (2020) discuss how failure to retain and promote BIPOC psychiatrists to the highest leadership levels results in lack of role-modeling and belonging.

In parallel, psychiatry training programs face challenges as they attempt to update their curriculums to more effective ones. In the latter half of the 20th century, a focus on cultural competence has transformed into cultural humility and sensitivity, as well as increasing recognition of the importance of structural competence.[15] To understand the many challenges faced by BIPOC trainees, training directors and supervisors must engage in self-education to recognize the impact that structural racism and implicit bias have in their institutions, and simultaneously, how these impact their ability to recruit and retain BIPOC candidates. The Cultural Formulation Interview chapter highlights the importance of focusing on these issues clinically and in the workplace.[16] That said, the field of psychiatry—and the use of the DSM in particular—perpetuates racist narratives about certain communities.[17] This reality is a barrier to recruiting diverse trainees.

Accreditation Council for Graduate Medical Education (ACGME) requirements in psychiatric training reflect this value and place increasing importance on workforce diversity and training of psychiatrists to become capable of caring for patients from diverse backgrounds. These guidelines require that trainees demonstrate competency in the areas of professionalism, patient care, and procedural skills.[18] Programs must also be careful not to blindly assume that pairing trainees with culturally congruent patients will always lead to better clinical outcomes. Rodriguez and colleagues[19] offer a vivid portrayal of the clinical challenges that can occur when a trainee and patient come from the same background and offer useful strategies for supervisors to consider when working with trainees of cultural backgrounds other than their own.

DISCUSSION
Recruitment Strategies

Pipeline within the same university

The Liaison Committee on Medical Education at the American Association of Medical Colleges has encouraged medical schools to become more racially and ethnically diverse throughout the past decade.[20] The encouragement has resulted in a more significant number of URM medical students whom psychiatry residency programs can recruit from their own institutions and beyond. Prior research has shown that connecting with a medical school's diversity office, psychiatry student interest group, and URM affinity groups can help recruit diverse applicants.[21,22]

However, the recruitment pipeline is not limited to the medical school affiliated with a residency program. More attention should be dedicated to students at earlier stages of training who are not yet in medical school, but who have expressed interest in the health sciences. For example, a case study by UCLA's Psychiatry Residency Program found that there is a missed opportunity to connect with premedical students who identify as URM. Psychiatry residency programs should build and leverage relationships with local high schools and community college programs to inspire interest in prospective trainees.[21] This would enable residency programs to showcase opportunities within the field of psychiatry and begin mentoring URM students at an early age.

Outreach to Historically Black Colleges and Universities and other universities

In addition to internal pipeline programs, strategic recruitment at Historically Black Colleges and Universities (HBCUs) can help increase diversity in graduate medical education.[23] For example, HBCUs only account for 2.6% of all medical students[24]; however, 15% of Black medical students attend HBCUs. The sizable Black population at these institutions represents a valuable opportunity to recruit individuals who are underrepresented in medicine.

In addition, HBCUs have set a high standard for diversifying academic medicine at all stages of training. A phenomenon known as the "*HBCU Medical School Effect*" describes how the number of Black medical students is positively related to the number of Black faculty and department chairs at an institution.[25] Although this piece is focused on diversifying the psychiatric workforce through training; to achieve that goal, we must diversify all levels of academic psychiatry. HBCUs have developed a successful model for increasing representation in academic medicine.[25] Psychiatry residency programs at other institutions would benefit from collaborating with and learning from HBCUs, and specifically recruiting medical students from these rich medical schools.

Selection: holistic review

A holistic review of residency applications is a method that residency programs can use to diversify their selection process.[23,26] This approach considers the totality of an individual's lived experiences in concert with their academic achievements.[23,27] This approach is also used to reduce reliance on measures tainted with bias, such as the USMLE Step 1.[28]

Regarding psychiatry, a recent study comparing holistic and traditional reviews found that individuals identifying as URM were greater than twice as likely to receive an interview under holistic criteria than conventional criteria.[28] One downside to conducting a holistic review is that it is typically more time-consuming than traditional methods, especially with more applications.[28,29] Therefore, successful implementation of holistic review will require that programs have more support.

Outreach to promising candidates
Programs can also increase the diversity of psychiatry trainees by actively and transparently conveying an interest in having a particular URM applicant train with them. The case study from UCLA recommended that having program directors and residents reach out to applicants after being interviewed can help establish connections.[21]

However, tailored outreach to URM applicants does not have to wait until an applicant has interviewed at a program. Programs can also conduct outreach throughout the application season, as evidenced by the Visiting Elective Scholarship Program (VESP) at UCSF. The VESP is a GME-wide initiative where URM students interested in particular specialties can participate in electives in the department of their choice.[30] Given the COVID-19 pandemic, the VESP program operated virtually in 2020, with the psychiatry department hosting multiple information sessions and recruitment events dedicated to URM students. In addition to VESP, many programs also host "Second Look" events that are specifically dedicated to giving URM applicants another opportunity to learn about a residency program.[31] These events typically focus on DEI-related initiatives and are meant to create a supportive community among prospective URM trainees.

Another strategy is to partner with community affinity groups. In 2020, the American Psychiatric Association's (APA) Black Caucus hosted a virtual event about DEI initiatives at 36 psychiatry residency programs for URM students. Seventy percent of the students reported that the event inspired them to learn more about a particular program.[32] Data have shown that applicants often find this type of outreach to be helpful. Residency programs might consider partnering with the APA Hispanic Caucus to hold a similar recruitment program early in the recruitment process.

Continuous quality improvement to measure the impact
As URM recruitment strategies are implemented, evaluating the programs' success in matching, and retaining URM applicants. We must identify measurable goals and metrics and be transparent about processes and progress. Evaluation measures are standard in residencies, but they are typically used to assess trainees' progress. For example, a 2007 study proposed a tripart paradigm of evaluation that focuses on the skills residents brought into the program ("before"), the experiences they had while training ("during"), and their achievements postgraduation ("after").[33] Training programs should measure dimensions including diversity, inclusion, and belonging and monitor performance from all residents, including those from minoritized identities. Metrics such as resident feedback from rotations, the ACGME survey, and the retention of faculty are ways to measure and monitor performance over time. We suggest taking an intersectional approach—specifically reviewing the intersection of gender identity and race/ethnicity—in evaluating trainees and faculty across their career trajectory. A similar framework could evaluate the success of a residency program's URM recruitment. By comparing a program's initial URM diversity, feedback from applicants who experience DEI programming, and the URM representation in a program's matriculating class, programs can identify what strategies helped them achieve their DEI metrics and which methods fell short. Ultimately, the qualitative and quantitative data collected,[33] can help continuously improve URM recruitment throughout the life of the residency program.

Retention Strategies to Promote Inclusion and Belonging

Create a supportive and inclusive environment
To increase diversity in residency programs, training directors need to implement strategies to retain our underrepresented trainees. Training directors need to consider the

climate of the residency training program and create supporting inclusive environments where trainees can thrive. Inclusion and belonging are critical for career satisfaction. Diversity without inclusion or belonging may lead to decreased well-being, increased burnout, and attrition.[34] Community building is one way to increase inclusion and belonging. Group activities, gatherings, and wellness events can build community. Community affinity groups began as race-based employee forums in corporate environments in response to the social conflict in the 1960s.[35] Today, community affinity groups go beyond race, they are meetings in which participants gather based on a particular social identity to discuss related personal experiences.[35] Community affinity groups can be centered around a shared identity or interest—and can create a community and mutual support for URM trainees.[36] In programs where there are small numbers of URM trainees, consider starting a joint community affinity group for URM trainees across all trainees in the institution. For example, Columbia University Medical School has formed a GME diversity council for resident members from any department.

In addition, trainee development programs through national organizations can provide additional support, mentorship, sponsorship, and belonging. The APA Minority Fellowship Programs are one such example. Regional and national meetings provide an opportunity to share experiences with other URM peers, get to know and spend time with URM faculty mentors. Such models may be limited in the trainees' home institution.

Increase role models

BIPOC trainees need to see URM role models at all aspects of the academic hierarchy, including in senior leadership roles. In addition to role models, ongoing mentorship, career development, and sponsorship are essential. Mentoring does not have to be from URM faculty only; mentoring from both URM faculty and non-URM faculty is valuable. All faculty should have required training in microaggressions, upstander skills, and mentoring people from backgrounds other than their own.[37,38] Mentors give advice and feedback while sponsors are in positions of power and use their influence and networks to create opportunities for others. Sponsorship—where people of power talk about a trainee and provide opportunities—is often missing in URM trainees' careers. Training programs should intentionally match URM trainees with sponsors or provide sponsoring opportunities by connecting the trainees to local, regional, and national leaders who can help to provide additional career guidance and recommend opportunities.[39] Notably, to reduce minority tax (see the following section), these URM role models should be compensated in some form (eg, relief from clinical duties, financially).

Decrease the minority tax

Several prominent underrepresented physicians have written about leaving academic medicine and organized psychiatry.[40,41] Problems such as structural and interpersonal racism and discrimination lead to URM faculty feeling they have to constantly prove their value and ability, distracting them from more meaningful activities. The "minority tax" of increased expectations for work that is not compensated or rewarded, including committee work, diversity-related institutional efforts, extra clinical assignments, voluntary community assignments, and mentoring, is commonly seen in URM trainees and faculty in academia. This tax contributes to burnout and poor retention of our diverse workforce.[42]

Faculty training in interpersonal and structural racism and response to bias

URM trainees experience microaggression frequently, up to 75% in some samples.[43] Microaggressions and other forms of racism and bias may lead to feelings of isolation, decreased self-esteem, poor mental and physical health, and burnout.[43] Recent data from ACGME reveal that Black, Asian, and Latinx trainees get dismissed from training programs at higher rates than White trainees.[44] Although the reasons for dismissal are unknown, bias is likely one of the drivers. In addition, in a recent review of over 30,000 medical students responding to the Association of American Medical Colleges (AAMC) Graduation Questionnaire, administered to graduating students at all 140 medical schools, URM student's disproportionality reporting perceiving a lack of respect for diversity among faculty.[45] Training directors need to be aware of the "hidden curriculum (knowledge not explicitly stated)," which trainees learn by watching the faculty and the institution. Separate care systems and under-resourced care for patients from community populations in contract to the faculty practice send a message to trainees. In addition, trainees are overhearing disparaging comments toward patients and trainees of color and are experiencing and often witnessing bias toward patients and trainees of color. Faculty development in structural and interpersonal racism to help faculty recognize bias is essential. Skill development such as upstander skills can help to change the culture. Senior leadership involvement and support of such faculty development are vital to model the necessary culture change.

The Training Itself: Opportunities for Intervention and Innovation

Structural competency built into the organization

Psychiatry training programs are at a critical juncture to respond to both the response to the COVID-19 and racism pandemics. Through crises emerges opportunities to meet the needs of our current cultural landscape. In recent decades, psychiatry training has shifted from focusing on cultural competence and characteristics of different social groups/identities toward a holistic frame through structural competency. Structural competency serves as a paradigm shift in understanding health and health disparities by critically examining the structural factors that impede well-being.[15] The approach guides providers to look beyond patient symptomatology and explore the social determinants of health also influencing the clinical encounter.[15] Competency, understood through the lens of cultural humility—an openness to continued self-reflection and learning.

Metzl and Hansen[15] describe structural competency training as composed of 5 skill sets: (1) recognizing the structures that shape clinical interactions (eg, economic, sociopolitical, and physical forces); (2) developing an extraclinical language of structure (eg, intersection of social structures and biology); (3) rearticulating "cultural" presentations in structural terms (eg, inclusion of structural forces and impacting care); (4) observing and imagining structural intervention (eg, consideration of methods to address structural health concerns); and (5) developing structural humility (eg, commitment to continued growth and awareness of limitations in examination of structural forces). Structural competency training moves providers from a purely diagnostic focus to more sophisticated conceptualizations that expand the clinical picture in the clinical environment. Considerations may include other relevant factors in care, such as the ability to afford medications, transportation to and from the appointment, and access to safe housing, to name a few. Our ability to see patients beyond individual characteristics to the larger social and societal structures they inhabit increases our ability to provide high-quality, patient-centered care. There is a robust Web site created by leaders in the field available for readers.[46]

In planning psychiatry training program curricula, training directors should consider an approach to building structural competency that provides continued exposure and increased complexity of experience over time. There is great benefit in repeated exposures to content regarding diversity and social inequities rather than singular or stand-alone training.[47] An ideal training model includes introspective awareness through cultural competency (eg, implicit bias, patient/provider communication) and a broader societal understanding by examining political, social, institutional, and economic factors.[15]

A developmental model allows for the inclusion of lower to higher experiences appropriate for the current level of training.[48] For instance, a developmental model may start with a focus on cultural self-awareness (implicit bias) and eventually move toward advocacy and action (participation in policy development). Like the structural competency training described earlier, such training is more effective when focusing on both awareness and skills.[47] One such example of a relevant tool for this is the "Structural Vulnerability Assessment," a screening instrument used to identify structural obstacles and inform resources and advocacy required to prevent poor health outcomes.[49] The answer to the screening question *"Do the places where you spend your time each day feel safe and healthy?"* can lead to the immediate consideration of needed resources or advocacy needed to obtain resources for vulnerable trainees.[49] The structural competency approach has also been described in relation to lesbian, gay, bisexual, transgender, gender nonconforming, and those with differences in sex development.[50] Although much of the initial training in structural competency may be didactic through understanding systemic forces, integrating opportunities for modeling action-oriented interventions expands this work from merely academic to transformative through advocacy.[51] As more psychiatry training programs seek to adopt structural competency training as part of their programs, psychiatry and national training organizations (e.g., AADPRT) must also provide continuing education and support for training directors to be sucessful in change managment. Many training directors are finding their trainees are more knowledgable on topics related to experiences of racism, discrimination, and health disparities. Psychiatry would benefit from a critical examination of training to move toward adopting a national diversity, equity, and inclusion curriculum setting standards and competiences for psychiatry.

Advocacy to promote antiracism

In adopting a structural competency model, we would be remiss not to consider how psychiatrists can effectively be advocates, particularly in addressing racism both within and outside of their organization. Kirmayer, Kronick, and Rousseau[51] posit that advocacy is, in fact, a core competency in psychiatry. For instance, a key competency in the University of California San Francisco (UCSF) Psychiatry HEAL Fellowship in Global Mental Health is engagement in the health system by way of evaluating health programs, engagement with local leaders/groups, and developing interventions with local partners.[52] The training program provides an ideal environment in which training faculty can model skills in advocacy and provide opportunities to put learning into action. Understandably many psychiatry faculty and residents are concerned that getting involved in advocacy means getting engaged in politics or working outside of one's scope. The reality is that the structural competency lens puts psychiatrists in an ideal position to understand the forces impacting those they serve and represent those interests on their behalf.

In developing advocacy skills, it is essential to model the different ways and levels one may advocate.[51] Kirmayer and colleagues outline 3 levels of advocacy: (1) recognizing and understanding the structural determinants of health and incorporating this knowledge into professional education, clinical practice, and community intervention; (2) supporting coalitions and collective action that aim to change policy and practice; and (3) initiating, mobilizing, and organizing, action to challenge social injustices.

Putting this into context, we want to understand the systemic factors compounding one's experience of depression, such as racism and discrimination. Still, we also seek to create more resources to reduce those factors that impact this individual and the broader community.

There is precedence for advocacy to be part of clinical training through community treatment teams identifying how systemic factors impact mental illness or developing a policy advocacy program where residents learned to draft bills enacted into law.[53] Although many URM residents may find themselves drawn to this work, White-identified faculty and residents must be encouraged to stretch the boundaries of their comfort zone toward incorporating advocacy as part of their psychiatry professional identity.

Promoting equal access to research

Despite many clinical programs focus on improving recruitment and retention of URM applicants, research training programs are another key area for growth. A structural competency approach to psychiatry training also requires a shift in the training and focus beyond predominately disease-focused research in White populations. Research is a critical component in developing needed interventions from science to practice and can help inform policy changes. Unfortunately, because of several factors, including mistreatment in health care and research, many marginalized communities are often not included or included in such small samples as to limit interpretation. There is a need to develop research programs that can address factors limiting participation, and that are able to effectively link outcomes to practice.[54]

One such approach to consider toward this effort is community-based participatory research (CBPR), which centers on the experience of the community studied at every facet of the research design.[54] CBPR builds on traditional approaches to soliciting research participants by going directly to the community studied to invite them into the process of creating the study rather than eliciting research participation without such investment.[55] The power of providing training opportunities in CBPR is that residents become more knowledgeable about the communities they serve (thus impacting clinical care outcomes), and through research, are better equipped to ask the right questions—questions that speak to the experience of the community. Moore and colleagues[54] proposed a model for equitable analysis including the following steps: (1) identify population or community of focus, (2) build relationships with community or patient leaders, (3) community engagement, (4) develop research questions and design, (5) data analysis and interpretation, (6) implementation and scaling of interventions, and (7) accountability. Training directors should seek to provide explicit training on this model in all psychiatry research training programs.

In addition, training directors should be mindful of the implicit bias that can lie in the types of research projects that are funded by large organizations, including NIH.[56] Institutions should consider building internal funding sources to support trainees interested in research on antiracism, health inequities, and structural determinants of health.

SUMMARY

The COVID-19 pandemic and murder of Mr George Floyd served as catalysts for examining antiracism efforts in psychiatry training programs and health care systems. Our recruitment and retention of Black, Indigenous, and other racial/ethnic minority psychiatry trainees has not met the demand for care and does not represent the communities served. Training directors at a critical juncture in creating systemic changes to recruitment, retention, policies, and curricular competencies to address ongoing inequities and disparities in health care. In this piece, we describe several strategies and considerations for training directors in supporting a diverse psychiatric workforce. Specifically, we describe strategies to improve recruitment including the development of intentional recruitment pipelines at universities, outreach to minority-serving universities, and examination of selection strategies to reduce bias are essential to increasing URM enrollment in psychiatry training programs. We also describe methods to retain trainees is through the creation of community affinity group spaces, and structured opportunities and mentorship with URM faculty. In general, we recommend that training programs move beyond cultural factors to examine how structural forces impact the experience of health care. Training curriculums should include a focus on structural competency, provide opportunities to engage in advocacy, and the development of research centered on participation of the communities of interest.

CLINICS CARE POINTS

Recommendation for Psychiatry Training Programs
- Recruitment
  - Bolster pipeline within your university (premedical students), local community colleges, and high schools
  - Create opportunities for interested BIPOC students to visit (eg, second visit, elective rotations)
  - Outreach to HBCUs and other institutions with high BIPOC enrollment
  - Partner with affinity groups within the APA for outreach
  - Holistic Review and ensure adequate support for successful implementation
  - Direct outreach to promising candidates
  - Continuous quality improvement to distill essential elements for successful recruitment
- Retention
  - Promote a supportive and inclusive environment, including implementation of community affinity groups.
  - Increase number of BIPOC role models for mentorship and sponsorship, but provide funding for this to decrease minority tax
  - Ensure that all faculty receive regular training in bias and allyship, and upstander behavior
  - Institute feedback mechanisms (quantitative and qualitative) and develop metrics to track progress over time
- Training
  - Include training in cultural competence, cultural humility, and structural competency
  - Provide opportunities for trainees to engage in advocacy as part of their curriculum, through modeling, and incorporation in training rotations
  - Develop trainee skills in conducting research centered on participation of the communities of interest.
  - Build internal funding structures to support research in antiracism, health inequities, and social determinants of health

DISCLOSURE

The authors have nothing to disclose.

REFERENCES

1. Frey WH. The nation is diversifying even faster than predicted, according to new census data. Brookings Institute; 2020. https://www.brookings.edu/research/new-census-data-shows-the-nation-is-diversifying-even-faster-than-predicted/.

2. Tamir C, Budiman A, Noe-Bustamante L, et al. Facts about the U.S. Black population. 2021. Available at;. https://www.pewresearch.org/social-trends/fact-sheet/facts-about-the-us-black-population/. Accessed August 2, 2021.

3. Wilson V. People of color will be a majority of the American working class in 2032. Economic Policy Institute 2016;9:1–27. https://www.epi.org/publication/the-changing-demographics-of-americas-working-class/#epi-toc-2.

4. FitzGerald C, Hurst S. Implicit bias in healthcare professionals: a systematic review. BMC Med Ethics 2017;18(1):1–18.

5. Alsan M, Garrick O, Graziani G. Does diversity matter for health? Experimental evidence from Oakland. Am Econ Rev 2019;109(12):4071–111.

6. Huerto R, Lindo E. Minority patients benefit from having minority doctors, but that's a hard match to make. University of Michigan Health 2020;. https://labblog.uofmhealth.org/rounds/minority-patients-benefit-from-having-minority-doctors-but-thats-a-hard-match-to-make-0.

7. Moran M. Psychiatry residency match numbers climb again after unprecedented year in medical education. 2021. Available at: https://psychnews.psychiatryonline.org/doi/10.1176/appi.pn.2021.5.27. Accessed August 2, 2021.

8. American Psychiatric Association. 2019 Resident/Fellow Census. 2020. Available at: https://www.psychiatry.org/File%20Library/Residents-MedicalStudents/Residents/APA-Resident-Census-2019.pdf. Accessed August 2, 2021.

9. Lee S. Racial disparities lead to poor mental health care for Black Americans. 2020. Available at: https://www.verywellmind.com/racial-disparities-mental-health-5072490. Accessed August 2, 2021.

10. Lin L, Stamm K, Christidis P. How diverse is the psychology workforce? Monitor Psychol 2018;49(2):19.

11. American Association of Medical Colleges. 2019 report on residents executive summary. 2019. Available at: https://www.aamc.org/data-reports/students-residents/interactive-data/report-residents/2019/executive-summary. Accessed August 2, 2021.

12. Hanson M. Average medical school debt. 2021. Available at: https://educationdata.org/average-medical-school-debt. Accessed August 2, 2021.

13. Molina MF, Landry AI, Chary AN, et al. Addressing the elephant in the room: microaggressions in medicine. Ann Emerg Med 2020;76(4):387–91.

14. Jordan A, Shim RS, Rodriguez CI, et al. Psychiatry Diversity Leadership in Academic Medicine: Guidelines for Success. Am J Psychiatry 2021;178(3):224–8.

15. Metzl JM, Hansen H. Structural competency: theorizing a new medical engagement with stigma and inequality. Social Sci Med 2014;103:126–33.

16. Lewis-Fernandez R, Aggarwal NK, Hinton L, et al. DSM-5® handbook on the cultural formulation interview. Arlington, VA: American Psychiatric Pub; 2016.

17. Medlock MM, Shtasel D, Trinh N-HT, et al. Racism and psychiatry: contemporary issues and interventions. Cham, Switzerland: Humana Press; 2019.

18. Accreditation Council for Graduate Medical Education. ACGME Program Requirements for Graduate Medical Education in Psychiatry. 2020. Available at: https://www.acgme.org/globalassets/pfassets/programrequirements/400_psychiatry_2020.pdf].

19. Rodriguez CI, Cabaniss DL, Arbuckle MR, et al. The role of culture in psychodynamic psychotherapy: parallel process resulting from cultural similarities between patient and therapist. Am J Psychiatry 2008;165(11):1402–6.

20. Richman EE, Ku BS, Cole AG. Advocating for underrepresented applicants to psychiatry: perspectives on recruitment. Am J Psychiatry Residents' J 2019; 14(2):2–4.

21. Pierre JM, Mahr F, Carter A, et al. Underrepresented in medicine recruitment: rationale, challenges, and strategies for increasing diversity in psychiatry residency programs. Acad Psychiatry 2017;41(2):226–32.

22. Brenner AM, Balon R, Coverdale JH, et al. Psychiatry workforce and psychiatry recruitment: two intertwined challenges41. Academic Psychiatry; 2017. p. 202–6.

23. Rohrbaugh RM, DeJong SM. The role of the program director in supporting diversity, equity, and inclusion. Academic Psychiatry; 2022. p. 264–8.

24. Yancy CW, Bauchner H. Diversity in medical schools—need for a new bold approach. JAMA 2021;325(1):31–2.

25. Rodríguez JE, López IA, Campbell KM, et al. The role of historically black college and university medical schools in academic medicine. J Health Care Poor Underserved 2017;28(1):266–78.

26. Aibana O, Swails JL, Flores RJ, et al. Bridging the gap: holistic review to increase diversity in graduate medical education. Acad Med 2019;94(8):1137–41.

27. Ross DA. The match: magic versus machines. J Graduate Med Edu 2019;11(3):274–6.

28. Barceló NE, Shadravan S, Wells CR, et al. Reimagining merit and representation: promoting equity and reducing bias in GME through holistic review. Acad Psychiatry 2021;45(1):34–42.

29. Walaszek A. Keep calm and recruit on: residency recruitment in an era of increased anxiety about the future of psychiatry. Acad Psychiatry 2017;41(2):213–20.

30. University of California San Francisco Medical Education. Visiting elective scholarship. 2021. Available at: https://meded.ucsf.edu/residents-clinical-fellows/gme-resident-and-fellow-resources/diversity-gme/visiting-elective-scholarship#WHO-CAN-APPLY. Accessed August 6, 2021.

31. University of California San Francisco Graduate Medical Education. UCSF GME Handbook for Holistic Review and Best Practices for Enhancing Diversity in Residency and Fellowship Programs. 2021. Available at: https://medschool.ucsf.edu/about/diversity/differences-matter/action-groups/focus-area-2-climate-recruitment.

32. Ojo E, Hairston D. Recruiting underrepresented minority students into psychiatry residency: a virtual diversity initiative45. Academic Psychiatry; 2021. p. 440–4.

33. Durning SJ, Hemmer P, Pangaro LN. The structure of program evaluation: an approach for evaluating a course, clerkship, or components of a residency or fellowship training program. Teach Learn Med 2007;19(3):308–18.

34. Gonzaga AMR, Appiah-Pippim J, Onumah CM, et al. A framework for inclusive graduate medical education recruitment strategies: meeting the ACGME standard for a diverse and inclusive workforce. Acad Med 2020;95(5):710–6.

35. Douglas PH. Affinity groups: Catalyst for inclusive organizations. Employment Relations Today 2008;34(4):11–8.

36. Tauriac JJ, Kim GS, Lambe Sariñana S, et al. Utilizing affinity groups to enhance intergroup dialogue workshops for racially and ethnically diverse students. J Specialists Group Work 2013;38(3):241–60.

37. Plews-Ogan ML, Bell TD, Townsend G, et al. Acting Wisely: Eliminating Negative Bias in Medical Education—Part 2: How Can We Do Better? Acad Med 2020;95(12S):S16–22.

38. Haynes-Baratz MC, Metinyurt T, Li YL, et al. Bystander training for faculty: a promising approach to tackling microaggressions in the academy. N Ideas Psychol 2021;63:100882.

39. Alves-Bradford J-M, Trinh N-H, Bath E, et al. Mental health equity in the twenty-first century: setting the stage. Psychiatr Clin 2020;43(3):415–28.

40. Blackstock U. Why Black doctors like me are leaving faculty positions in academic medical centers. 2020. Available at: https://www.statnews.com/2020/01/16/black-doctors-leaving-faculty-positions-academic-medical-centers/. Accessed August 12, 2021.

41. Shim RS. Structural racism is why I'm leaving organized psychiatry. 2020. Available at: https://www.statnews.com/2020/07/01/structural-racism-is-why-im-leaving-organized-psychiatry/. Accessed August 12, 2021.

42. Rodríguez JE, Campbell KM, Pololi LH. Addressing disparities in academic medicine: what of the minority tax? BMC Med Educ 2015;15(1):6.

43. Sandoval RS, Afolabi T, Said J, et al. Building a tool kit for medical and dental students: addressing microaggressions and discrimination on the wards. MedEdPORTAL 2020;16:1–12.

44. Vela MB, Chin MH, Peek ME. Keeping our promise—supporting trainees from groups that are underrepresented in medicine. N Engl J Med 2021;385(6):487–9.

45. Weiss J, Balasuriya L, Cramer LD, et al. Medical students' demographic characteristics and their perceptions of faculty role modeling of respect for diversity. JAMA Netw Open 2021;4(6):e2112795.

46. Structural competency. Structural competency: new medicine for inequalities that are making us sick. structuralcompetency.org.

47. Bezrukova K, Spell CS, Perry JL, et al. A meta-analytical integration of over 40 years of research on diversity training evaluation. Psychol Bull 2016;142(11):1227.

48. Jones JM, Sander JB, Booker KW. Multicultural competency building: Practical solutions for training and evaluating student progress. Train Edu Prof Psychol 2013;7(1):12.

49. Bourgois P, Holmes SM, Sue K, et al. Structural vulnerability: operationalizing the concept to address health disparities in clinical care. Acad Med 2017;92(3):299.

50. Donald CA, DasGupta S, Metzl JM, et al. Queer frontiers in medicine: a structural competency approach. Acad Med 2017;92(3):345–50.

51. Kirmayer LJ, Kronick R, Rousseau C. Advocacy as key to structural competency in psychiatry. JAMA psychiatry 2018;75(2):119–20.

52. Buzza C, Fiskin A, Campbell J, et al. Competencies for global mental health: developing training objectives for a post-graduate fellowship for psychiatrists. Ann Glob Health 2018;84(4):717.

53. Hansen H, Braslow J, Rohrbaugh RM. From cultural to structural competency—training psychiatry residents to act on social determinants of health and institutional racism. JAMA Psychiatry 2018;75(2):117–8.

54. Moore Q, Tennant PS, Fortuna LR. Improving research quality to achieve mental health equity. Psychiatr Clin 2020;43(3):569–82.

55. Collins SE, Clifasefi SL, Stanton J, et al. Community-based participatory research (CBPR): towards equitable involvement of community in psychology research. Am Psychol 2018;73(7):884.

56. Hoppe TA, Litovitz A, Willis KA, et al. Topic choice contributes to the lower rate of NIH awards to African-American/black scientists. Sci Adv 2019;5(10):eaaw7238.

Enhancing the Pipeline for a Diverse Workforce

Quinn Capers IV, MD[a],*, Lia Thomas, MD[b]

KEYWORDS

- Pipeline • Underrepresented minority • Bias • Diversity • Disparities
- Structural racism • Hispanic • Black

KEY POINTS

- The lack of diversity in the physician workforce is a multifactorial problem with several potential culprits.
- Structural racism and inequities in housing, income, and education put minority children who aspire to advanced degrees at a competitive disadvantage.
- This disadvantage can be attenuated with "pipeline" programs that expose children to the medical profession early and provide academic support to high school and college students.
- Bias mitigation and recruitment at the "deep pipeline" of young students, the "intermediate pipeline" of college students, and the "end game" of selection processes is critical.
- Many academic medical centers, government-funded programs, and volunteer organizations are currently working to enhance the educational pipeline with well-prepared minority students. These programs need continued support.

INTRODUCTION: THE PROBLEM

The lack of diversity in the physician workforce in the United States is a long-standing problem that negatively impacts health care equity, medical education, and the cultural competence of all health care workers. The argument that diversity in medicine will enhance health care for all populations is easy to make, with evidence showing that physicians who train in racially diverse environments rate themselves as more comfortable treating patients of different backgrounds,[1] minority patients are more likely to comply with recommendations for preventive services and treatments such as vaccines and heart surgery when recommended by race-concordant physicians,[2,3]

This article originally appeared in *Psychiatric Clinics*, Volume 45 Issue 2, June 2022.

[a] Department of Medicine, University of Texas Southwestern Medical Center, 5323 Harry Hines Boulevard, Dallas, TX 75390, USA; [b] Department of Psychiatry, University of Texas Southwestern Medical Center, 5323 Harry Hines Boulevard, Dallas, TX 75390, USA
* Corresponding author.
E-mail address: Quinn.capers@UTSouthwestern.edu
Twitter: @DrQuinnCapers4 (Q.C.); @DrLiaT1 (L.T.)

Child Adolesc Psychiatric Clin N Am 33 (2024) 71–76
https://doi.org/10.1016/j.chc.2023.06.008
1056-4993/24/

Black physicians are least likely of all physician groups to harbor negative implicit racial biases about other races,[4] medical research performed by racially diverse teams is cited more often than research by less diverse teams,[5] minority physicians are more likely than others to choose to serve underserved and disadvantaged communities,[6] and women physicians may outperform men when following evidence-based guidelines to the benefit of their patients.[7]

Because data indicate that more minorities and women in medicine will enhance health care quality for all and may well save more lives, the lack of diversity in medicine should be addressed with urgency. However, structural racism such as inequities in housing, employment, and access to well-funded, high-performing schools results in a significant shortage of Hispanic, Black, Native American, Native Pacific Islander, or Native Alaskan students well prepared to study medicine.[8] These individuals are not only underrepresented in the medical profession but also are in short supply at key points in the medical school pipeline. Thus, strategies to enhance diversity in medicine must include actions to enrich the educational pipeline with well-prepared minority students.

It is useful to consider diversity enhancement in medicine in 3 stages: the "deep pipeline" of high school and pre–high school students, the "intermediate pipeline" of college and medical students, and the "end game," or selection processes into medical school or residency/fellowship training programs. Success promoting compositional diversity at one stage facilitates success in the other 2. It is important that medical schools, typically the site where the "end game" processes play out, take an active role in developing pipelines of diverse individuals. Traditionally, institutions wait for minority individuals to complete medical training before attempting to diversify their faculty rosters and training programs. This passive approach has not yielded results in over a century of medical education. Academic medical departments and centers that defend their lack of diversity by stating "We could not find qualified candidates" should be challenged with the question "What are you doing to develop a pipeline of diverse individuals in your specialty so that 10 years from now that statement will no longer be true?"

"Deep PIPELINE"

Although research has shown that postbaccalaureate programs have been quite successful at preparing college graduates from minority and disadvantaged backgrounds to pursue medicine,[9] educational literature suggests an attrition of minority students much earlier in the pipeline. In a cohort study of nearly 25,000 White, Black, Asian, and Hispanic children followed from the eighth to the twelfth grade, Black boys and Hispanic girls were the most likely to drop aspirations to attend college or graduate/professional school during the study period.[10] These and other findings support the contention that outreach efforts to enhance diversity in medicine need to start much earlier than college.

Exposing children in the pre–high school and high school years to medicine as a career can be done by individual clinicians, school systems in partnerships with health care organizations or medical schools, or private or volunteer initiatives. Many medical schools have programs to expose minority children to careers in the health professions. Some examples of non–medical school programs that expose children to the health sciences include the following:

- Young Doctors DC (https://www.youngdoctorsdc.org) (Washington, DC-based program to mentor high school boys into health professions careers.)
- Young Physicians Initiative (ypiprogram.com) (Atlanta, GA-based program that provides interactive guidance to underserved middle school, high school, and college students interested in medical careers.)

- American College of Cardiology Young Scholars Program (https://www.acc.org/Membership/Sections-and-Councils/Academic-Cardiology-Section/Young-Scholars-Program): an initiative of the American College of Cardiology that aims to provide promising young high school and college students with an introduction to the field of cardiology and strengthen the pipeline of talent for the future.

Because the attrition of minority students aspiring to be doctors may start before or shortly after the eighth grade, we encourage medical schools to invite local elementary school children to visit their state-of-the-art clinical skills simulation centers for proctored experiences that explore medical procedures or cardiopulmonary resuscitation. Involving minority medical or health professions students as proctors in these activities can provide important role models for the children. It is widely accepted that for children in underrepresented minority groups, seeing Hispanic, Black, or Native American doctors is critically important for their self-esteem and confidence. Patching the "leaky pipeline" of talent at this early stage can provide more motivated, prepared students for the next stage.

INTERMEDIATE PIPELINE

Postbaccalaureate programs that prepare minority college students or recent graduates to successfully navigate the medical school application process are a great benefit to society. These programs go beyond traditional premed advising and offer a chance to study undergraduate or graduate-level courses. These programs can take place during the summer breaks or after receiving an undergraduate degree. All such programs aim to buttress academic skills to make students more competitive for medical school, with many including formal preparation for the Medical College Admissions Test. Examples include Georgetown University's GEMS program (GEMS Post-Baccalaureate Program | School of Medicine | Georgetown University) and Southern Illinois University's MEDPREP program (MEDPREP | SIU School of Medicine [siumed.edu]). A few medical school-run postbaccalaureate programs are linked to a guarantee of acceptance into the entering medical school class for students who meet prespecified academic performance targets. The latter are what many consider true "pipeline" programs. An example of this type of program is The Ohio State University's MEDPATH program (MEDPATH Program | Ohio State College of Medicine [osu.edu]).

THE "END GAME" (SELECTION PROCESSES)

The child from a minority or disadvantaged background who dreams of becoming a doctor faces nearly 2 decades of hurdles. Such children must navigate low expectations from teachers,[11,12] racial disparities in school discipline,[13] and a lower likelihood of being assigned to "gifted and talented" programs despite equivalent high grades.[14] These circumstances describe what has been called the "leaky pipeline" of talented minority students prepared to pursue medicine. A more accurate description would be that minority children are being actively extruded from the pipeline. When minority students persist despite these obstacles and emerge well prepared to study medicine, they face an additional, invisible hurdle: implicit racial bias among members of the medical school admissions committee.[15] This essay is principally about the importance of pipeline programs in diversifying medicine, but if that pipeline delivers aspiring physicians into a racially biased selection process, the result will be a "traffic pile-up" of talented individuals outside of our medical schools. Thus, it is important that transformative work on the deep and intermediate pipelines and the end game selection processes proceed simultaneously.

Holistic Review

Most medical school admissions committees have moved beyond relying solely on scholastic grades and standardized test scores as the sole criteria upon which to base selection. Although critical thinking and intelligence remain highly desirable traits in future doctors, many committees place an equal value on characteristics such as community service, leadership, communication skills, and the diversity of background and thought that the candidate brings. This "holistic review" of applicants has proved to be effective not only at diversifying student bodies but in enhancing individual and group student success.[16] Preliminary data indicate that following a holistic review strategy in graduate medical education selection processes can likewise promote diversity in residency training programs.[17]

Implicit Bias Mitigation

Implicit biases related to the race,[15] weight, and even perceived "attractiveness"[18] of medical school or residency/fellowship applicants may influence the selection processes of physicians in the United States. The authors believe it is important for individuals participating in selection committees to participate in exercises to identify and mitigate their own biases.[18,19] It can be argued that this should be done not only at the "end game" of undergraduate and graduate medical education selections but also by those making decisions on student progress at the deep and intermediate pipeline stages.

The Pipeline and the Psychiatric Workforce

All the aforementioned recommendations can and should be incorporated into strategies enhancing the psychiatric workforce. With regard to the deep pipeline, introduction of the concepts of mental health and wellness should be part of high school curricula with examples of how these concepts can turn into careers. Organized psychiatry could partner with school behavioral counselors to introduce students to the spectrum of mental health professionals. As many schools introduce social and emotional learning into curriculum, an exploration of the many fields in mental health could be introduced.

At the level of the intermediate pipeline, psychiatric practitioners and groups can reach out to premed societies at local colleges and offer clinical shadowing experiences or invite minority college students to professional meetings. In medical schools academic psychiatry departments typically interact with medical students via specialty interest groups. Intentional outreach to minority student organizations, such as the student national medical association, Latino medical student association, and others, can encourage minorities to consider the field. A regional program in the state of Texas was modestly successful at mentoring medical students to participate in academic psychiatry projects. If continued and duplicated, such programs could be expected to increase interest in training in psychiatry.

SUMMARY

The lack of diversity in the physician workforce is a multifactorial problem. From elementary school through college, students from minority or socioeconomically disadvantaged backgrounds achieve despite attending underresourced schools, facing low expectations from peers and teachers, and overcoming unconscious biases among decision makers. These and other obstacles lead to significant attrition of talent by the time cohorts prepare to apply to medical school. Pipeline initiatives that inspire and prepare applicants from groups underrepresented in medicine are needed to swell the ranks of diverse individuals entering our profession. Many informal "exposure" programs and formal pipeline programs are active across the nation and must proliferate and be supported while we continue to work to eliminate bias in the selection processes. Medicine will not reach its full potential until we welcome and leverage talent from all backgrounds and communities.

CLINICS CARE POINTS

- Physicians from Underrepresented groups (Hispanic, Black, Native American, Native Alaskan, Native Pacific Islander) are more likely than others to choose to serve underserved communities.

- Minority patients are more likely to comply with recommendations of race-concordant physicians

- Majority physicians who train in diverse environments are more comfortable treating minority patients

- Increasing the number of minority physicians and psychiatrists will require the proliferation and support of pipeline programs that prepare students to enter the medical profession

DISCLOSURE

The authors have no conflicts to disclose. There was no funding for this article.

REFERENCES

1. Saha S, Guiton G, Wimmers PF, et al. Student body raialracial and ethnic composition and diversity-related outcomes in US medical schools. JAMA 2008;300: 1135–45. https://doi.org/10.1001/jama.300.10.1135.
2. Alsan M, Garrick O, Grant G. Does diversity matter for health? Experimental evidence from Oakland. Am Econ Rev 2019;109:4071–111. https://doi.org/10.1257/aer.20181446.
3. Saha S, Beach MC. Impact of physician race on patient decision-making and ratings of physicians: a randomized experiment using video vignettes. J Gen Intern Med 2020;35:1084–91. https://doi.org/10.1007/s11606-020-05646-z.
4. Sabin J, Nosek BA, Greenwald A, et al. Physicians' implicit and explicit attitudes about race by MD race, ethnicity, and gender. J Health Care Poor Underserved 2009;20:896–913. https://doi.org/10.1353/hpu.0.0185.
5. AlShebli BK, Rahwan T, Woon WL. The preeminence of ethnic diversity in scientific collaboration. Nat Commun 2018;9:5163. https://doi.org/10.1038/s41467-018-07634-8.
6. Garcia AN, Kuo T, Arangua L, et al. Factors associated with medical school graduates' intention to work with underserved populations: policy implications for advancing workforce diversity. Acad Med 2018;93:82–9. https://doi.org/10.1097/ACM.0000000000001917.
7. Tsugawa Y, Jena AB, Figueroa JF, et al. Comparison of hospital mortality and readmission rates for Medicare patients treated by male vs female physicians. JAMA Intern Med 2017;177:206–13. https://doi.org/10.1001/jamainternmed.2016.787.
8. Dent RB, Vichare A, Casimir J. Addressing Structural Racism in the Health Workforce. Med Care 2021;59(Suppl 5):S409–12.

9. McDougle L, Way DP, Lee WK, et al. A National Long-term Outcomes Evaluation of U.S. Premedical Postbaccalaureate Programs Designed to Promote Health care Access and Workforce Diversity. J Health Care Poor Underserved 2015; 26(3):631–47.
10. Kao G, Tienda M. Educational aspirations of minority youth. Am J Educ 1998; 106(3):349–84. https://www.jstor.org/stable/1085583.
11. Teachers' implicit bias against black students starts in preschool, study finds | Race | The Guardian. Accessed October 28, 2021. https://www.theguardian. com/world/2016/oct/04/black-students-teachers-implicit-racial-bias-preschool-study.
12. The Power of Teacher Expectations - Education Next. Accessed October 28, 2021. https://www.educationnext.org/power-of-teacher-expectations-racial-bias-hinders-student-attainment/.
13. Riddle T, Sinclair S. Racial disparities in school-based disciplinary actions are associated with county-level rates of racial bias. PNAS Apr 2019;116(17): 8255–60.
14. Grissom JA, Redding C. Discretion and Disproportionality: Explaining the Under-representation of high-Achieving students of color in gifted programs. AERA Open 2016. https://doi.org/10.1177/2332858415622175.
15. Capers Q 4th, Clinchot D, McDougle L, et al. Implicit Racial Bias in Medical School Admissions. Acad Med 2017;92(3):365–9.
16. Urban Universities for Health. Holistic Admissions in the Health Professions. Available at: http://urbanuniversitiesforhealth.org/media/documents/Holistic_Admissions_in_the_Health_Professions.pdf. Accessed September 20, 2020.
17. Aibana O, Swails JL, Flores RJ, et al. Bridging the Gap: Holistic Review to In-crease Diversity in Graduate Medical Education. Acad Med 2019;94(8):1137–41.
18. Capers Q 4th. How Clinicians and Educators Can Mitigate Implicit Bias in Patient Care and Candidate Selection in Medical Education. ATS Sch 2020;1(3):211–7.
19. Harris TB, Mian A, Lomax JW, et al. The Texas regional psychiatry minority Mentor network: a regional effort to increase psychiatry's workforce diversity. Acad Psy-chiatry 2012;36:60–3.

The Role of the National Institute of Mental Health in Promoting Diversity in the Psychiatric Research Workforce

Lauren D. Hill, PhD[a], Shelli Avenevoli, PhD[b],
Joshua A. Gordon, MD, PhD[b],*

KEYWORDS

- Mental health research • Equity • Diversity and inclusion • Workforce development

KEY POINTS

- Diversity enhances the capacity to address complex problems.
- Significant systemic obstacles impede effort to ensure a diverse and inclusive mental health research workforce.
- Equitable funding decision processes, diversity-promoting training opportunities, and support for research in health disparities are 3 important steps to take to build a more diverse workforce.

The recent events of the COVID-19 pandemic and widespread video broadcasts and news reports of lethal attacks on African Americans by law enforcement have brought us to a pivotal moment in our shared history. The pandemic laid bare long-standing racial disparities in health, and the stress of both the pandemic and ongoing violence has disproportionately impacted the mental health of Black Americans and other racial and ethnic minority groups.[1] The long-standing imperative to achieve racial equity and to end structural racism has become more urgent than ever. This urgency has prompted reflection, discussion, and action at the National Institutes of Health (NIH) and the National Institute of Mental Health (NIMH). NIMH's mission is to transform the understanding and treatment of mental illnesses through basic and clinical research, paving the way for prevention, recovery, and cure. NIMH fulfills this mission through supporting and conducting research on mental illnesses and the underlying basic science of

This article originally appeared in *Psychiatric Clinics*, Volume 45 Issue 2, June 2022.
[a] Office for Disparities Research and Workforce Diversity, National Institute of Mental Health, National Institutes of Health, 31 Center Drive, MS2116, Bethesda, MD 20892-2116, USA;
[b] Office of the Director, National Institute of Mental Health, National Institutes of Health, 31 Center Drive, MS2116, Bethesda, MD 20892-2116, USA
* Corresponding author.
E-mail address: joshua.gordon@nih.gov

Child Adolesc Psychiatric Clin N Am 33 (2024) 77–86
https://doi.org/10.1016/j.chc.2023.06.009
1056-4993/24/Published by Elsevier Inc.

the brain and behavior, supporting the training of scientists to carry out basic and clinical mental health research, and communicating with scientists, patients, providers, and the public about the science of mental illnesses. To achieve this mission, NIMH needs to ensure that the brightest ideas are examined by the most capable scientists who provide a variety of perspectives on the complex problems we strive to solve. Supporting a diverse mental health research workforce is therefore an integral component of achieving the NIMH mission. Such efforts do not, however, occur in a vacuum. A long history of racist laws, principles, policies, and practices impact nearly all aspects of society in the United States, including education, science, medicine, and academia. Structural racism has negatively impacted equity, diversity, and inclusion in the mental health research workforce.[2] The causes are complex and manifold, and the strategies to address them must also be multifaceted.

Accordingly, achieving a diverse, equitable, and inclusive mental health research workforce will require a sustained, purposeful, and multidimensional effort. To build such an effort requires attention to 3 key areas: ensuring a just and equitable funding process; building a diverse workforce through training; and supporting research in health disparities and other understudied areas that are often the focus of scientists from underrepresented and marginalized groups.

UNDERSTANDING AND PROMOTING DIVERSITY IN THE SCIENTIFIC WORKFORCE

The NIMH research workforce benefits from the diversity of investigators from a variety of basic and applied behavioral health science disciplines, including, but not limited to, neuroscience, psychiatry, psychology, social work, and health services and implementation science. Unfortunately, the racial and ethnic composition of our workforce is not diverse enough to reap the full benefits of the life experiences and perspectives that scientists and trainees from diverse backgrounds bring to the research enterprise. Diversity enhances capacity to address complex problems. Research on corporate workgroups in business, economics, and technology demonstrates that diverse groups outperform homogeneous groups in a range of valuable outcomes.[3,4]

Compelling arguments have been made for the importance of racial and ethnic diversity in the larger psychiatric workforce, including improvements in medical education and the provision of health care services to diverse populations.[5] Promoting cultures of inclusion and diversity in medical education, psychiatry residency training, and psychiatric professional societies have been identified as important steps toward improving patients' health by embracing values that support health equity, reduce health care disparities, and enhance the cultural competency of the workforce overall.[6]

Obstacles to equity, diversity, and inclusion in psychiatry research include, but are not limited to, factors related to the culture of the research enterprise, including interpersonal, institutional, and structural factors. A necessary first step toward addressing these obstacles is acknowledging both the historical origins and the current consequences of a complex set of structural factors that has led to a research workforce that neither reflects the racial and ethnic diversity of the nation as a whole nor the diverse set of communities that workforce serves.[7] In January 2021, the American Psychiatric Association (APA) issued an apology to Black, Indigenous, and other People of Color (BIPOC) for its support of structural racism in psychiatry.[8] The apology and a historical addendum[9] acknowledged both actions and inactions on the part of the organization and its members that have resulted in harm to BIPOC individuals, patients, families, and APA members. Similar statements by Dr Francis Collins, Director of the NIH,[10] and by Dr Joshua Gordon, Director of the NIMH,[11] explicitly recognize the role that the NIH, NIMH, and others in the biomedical research field have played in perpetuating the structures that contribute to systemic racism and the need for concerted and persistent action to achieve a more equitable, diverse, and inclusive research enterprise.

Identification of structural and cultural practices and policies that pose barriers to equity, diversity, and inclusion in the scientific enterprise informs the development of practices and policies designed to dismantle those barriers. As stated above, these are complex and multifaceted, but among the barriers to be identified and addressed are biases in decision making about the merit and value of research applications, underrepresentation of racial and ethnic minority group members in the research workforce, and a historic marginalization of minority mental health and mental health disparities research.

ENSURING A JUST AND EQUITABLE FUNDING PROCESS

Despite its importance, efforts to build a diverse workforce can be thwarted by the cumulative actions of those who make decisions about admissions, recruitment, hiring, and promotion. Decisions about who receives admission to academic institutions or professional societies, promotion and tenure along the career pathway, advancement to positions of leadership, what research is worthy of support, and who gets to make those decisions reflect the implicit and explicit values and biases of the cultures in which the decisions are made; in this case within the scientific enterprise. These critical decisions directly impact education, opportunities, and career trajectories. Federal research grant funding frequently plays a role, often indirectly, in these consequential decisions. The availability of federal funds bolsters the infrastructure of research institutions, which in turn, plays a role in the number of research trainees and staff that can be supported, as well as the research resources available to both trainees and faculty members. NIH funding pays faculty and staff scientist salaries as well as trainee stipends, and grant support is often correlated with promotion and tenure trajectories.[12,13]

The landmark paper by Ginther and colleagues[14] impelled NIH to confront the finding that applications supporting Black principal investigators (PIs) were 10 percentage points less likely than those supporting White PIs to receive NIH research funding, even after controlling for educational background, country of origin, training, previous research awards, publication record, and employer characteristics. Other studies have followed, in attempts to understand factors that contribute to those racial disparities.[15–18] These disparities contribute further to inequality of opportunity for underrepresented scientists.

As noted above, it has been known for over a decade that applications with White PIs are funded at higher rates than those with PIs of color across the NIH. An analysis of more than 10 years' worth of NIMH R01 application data revealed that racial disparities in NIMH funding are equally profound.[19] Over the period from 2008 to 2018, only 11% of NIH applications supporting Black investigators were funded compared with 20% of applications supporting White investigators. A finer-grained analysis revealed disparities that disadvantage applications supporting Black investigators occurred at multiple steps throughout the NIMH funding process (**Fig. 1**). NIMH received fewer applications with Black PIs than without Black PIs, both in total number of applications (ratio of 1 application received with Black PIs for every 34 received without a Black PI) and in the number of applications per unique PI. Fewer applications with Black PIs were discussed by study sections, and those that were discussed were less likely

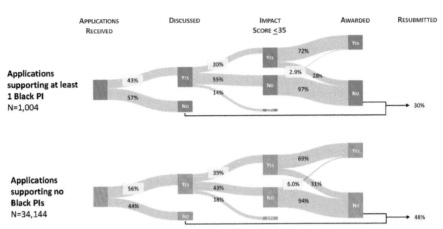

Fig. 1. Application review process: applications received, discussed, scored, awarded, and re-submitted supporting at least one Black PI and no Black applicants, 2008 to 2019. The percentage of applications that moved from one phase of the review process to the next is shown for those applications administered by NIMH supporting at least 1 Black PI and supporting no Black PIs. Applications with no information on race were excluded from this analysis (N = 2924). An Impact Score of 35 was chosen for the purpose of this analysis to identify those applications most likely to be considered for award, where the final overall impact scores range from 10 (high impact) through 90 (low impact). For more information on Impact Scores, see https://grants.nih.gov/grants/peer-review.htm. "OTH" represents those applications with no Impact Score or an Impact Score in a retired format. Less than 1% of applications that were not discussed received scores; for the sake of readability, these are not shown. Includes R01-equivalents, other Research Project Grants (RPGs), Cooperative Agreements and Center Grants, and Small Business Innovation Research/Small Business Technology Transfer (SBIR/STTR). Excludes training (training-related, fellowship and career development, Loan Repayment Program), Brain Research through Advancing Innovative Neurotechnologies (BRAIN) Initiative, Common Fund, NIH Blueprint for Neuroscience Research, NIH Helping to End Addiction Long-term SM Initiative (NIH HEAL Initiative SM), American Recovery and Reinvestment Act (ARRA), supplements, Resource Access Mechanism, and other activity codes, such as R13, SB1, SC1, SC2. Both new awards and continuations (as described at https://report.nih.gov/sites/report/files/docs/NIH%20Success%20Rate%20Definition%202018.pdf) are included for analysis. Applicants self-reported gender, race, and ethnicity when submitting their applications; for considerations relating to confidentiality, data security, and reporting, see https://grants.nih.gov/grants/collection-of-personal-demographic-data.htm and https://era.nih.gov/privacy-act-and-era.htm.

to receive a strong score. Finally, of those not receiving strong scores, fewer were funded.

These discrepancies strongly suggest a systemic bias that demands a multifaceted solution. At NIMH, several measures are being simultaneously undertaken to address the issue. First, the NIH's Center for Scientific Review and the review branch at NIMH have both redoubled efforts to enhance the diversity of review panels by increasing outreach and through targeted recruiting efforts to diversify the pool of prospective panel member candidates. Second, through the Brain Research through Advancing Innovative Neurotechnologies (BRAIN) Initiative, the NIMH and other NIH Institutes and Centers have begun to pilot a required, score-driving Plan for Enhancing Diverse Perspectives to be included in grant applications.[20] This pilot is being gradually expanded to additional applications. Third, we have ensured that the postreview decision-making process at NIMH takes into account the fact that diversity of scientific perspectives enhances our overall portfolio. Together, these efforts are aimed at ensuring that all applications, regardless of the PIs' backgrounds, have an equitable chance of success. So far, these early efforts seem to be having an effect: funding rates through Fiscal Year 2020 demonstrate a narrowing of the funding gaps between Black and White PIs (**Fig. 2**).

BUILDING A DIVERSE WORKFORCE THROUGH TRAINING

Building a diverse scientific workforce is an essential component of the NIMH mission to transform the understanding and treatment of mental illnesses. Nevertheless, our current mental health research workforce is lacking considerably in diversity. In 2020, for example, only 5% of PIs on grant applications to NIMH were Hispanic/Latino, and 3% were Black. One of the primary ways that NIMH has attempted to improve scientific workforce diversity is through research training opportunities for individuals from diverse backgrounds, with a particular emphasis on providing mentorship, research experience, and financial support during transitional career stages. A focus on career development supports a diverse pool of highly trained scientists prepared to

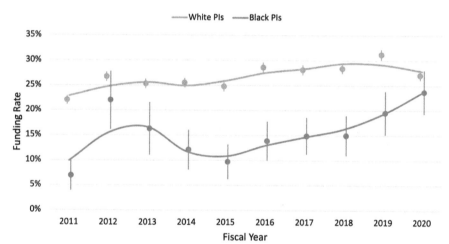

Fig. 2. NIMH funding rate among applications supporting White PIs and Black PIs, 2011 to 2020. Bars are standard errors of the funding rate reflecting statistical uncertainty. Smoothed curves reflect a weighted moving average using Loess regression. As described here, https://report.nih.gov/nihdatabook/category/22, "[f]unding rate is a person-based statistical that is calculated by the number of distinct funded investigators divided by the number of distinct funded and unfunded investigators in a given fiscal year, excluding applications withdrawn prior to review." Includes R01-equivalents, other Research Project Grants (RPGs), Cooperative Agreements and Center Grants, and SBIR/STTR. Excludes training (training-related, fellowship and career development, Loan Repayment Program), BRAIN Initiative, Common Fund, NIH Blueprint for Neuroscience Research, NIH HEAL Initiative SM, ARRA, supplements, Resource Access Mechanism, and other activity codes, such as R13, SB1, SC1, SC2. Both new awards and continuations (as described here, https://report.nih.gov/sites/report/files/docs/NIH%20Success%20Rate%20Definition%202018.pdf) are included for analysis. Applicants self-reported gender, race, and ethnicity when submitting their applications; for considerations relating to confidentiality, data security, and reporting, see https://grants.nih.gov/grants/collection-of-personal-demographic-data.htm and https://era.nih.gov/privacy-act-and-era.htm.

address research needs. A diversified portfolio that includes an assortment of training opportunities aims to ensure that we are reaching a wide variety of individuals, career pathways, and training institutions and are continually incorporating what we learn about critical points along the career pathway and individual and institutional challenges. NIMH participates in several new and long-standing funding opportunities and supplement programs that support individual investigators from diverse backgrounds at multiple stages of the career pathway: student, postdoctoral fellow, and early-stage investigator. These opportunities are described in later discussion, but please see https://www.nimh.nih.gov/funding/training for additional information.

For predoctoral students of diverse backgrounds, NIMH supports several individual awards focused on increasing research career preparedness, including the Ruth L. Kirschstein National Research Service Award (NRSA) Individual Predoctoral Fellowship to Promote Diversity in Health-Related Research (Parent F31–Diversity), the Mental Health Dissertation Research Grant to Increase Diversity (R36), and the NIH Blueprint Diversity Specialized Predoctoral to Postdoctoral Advancement in Neuroscience (D-SPAN) Award (F99/K00). The NRSA Diversity F31 supports individualized, mentored research training at any stage of predoctoral work. The R36 Mental Health Dissertation Grants are specifically intended to facilitate the completion of the dissertation and fill a gap in funding when institutional support typically wanes. The D-SPAN award is a more specialized program aimed at enhancing diversity in neuroscience. This 2-phased award enables completion of the doctoral dissertation as well as the transition to a neuroscience research postdoctoral position. Postdoctoral fellows from diverse backgrounds may be eligible for one of two K99/R00 awards that facilitate a timely transition from mentored, postdoctoral research positions to independent, research-intensive faculty positions: the Maximizing Opportunities for Scientific and Academic Independent Careers Postdoctoral Career Transition Award to Promote Diversity (K99/R00), and the BRAIN Initiative Advanced Postdoctoral Career Transition Award to Promote Diversity (K99/R00).

In addition to the individual awards described above, NIMH also supports institutional awards with the goal of diversifying its offerings and ensuring that training opportunities are available to a wide array of individuals across career stages. Examples include the NIH Blueprint for Neuroscience Research–ENDURE Undergraduate Program and the NIH Neuroscience Development for Advancing the Careers of a Diverse Research Workforce (R25) award. Both support neuroscience educational activities of those from diverse backgrounds. NIMH has more recently added support for mission-relevant scientific conferences that promote inclusion of women and individuals from underrepresented groups. Funds for Conference Grants (R13) to Promote Inclusion in the Research Workforce must be used to support conference attendance and specific programming events that enhance trainee learning, mentorship, inclusion, and professional development.

Another mainstay of NIMH workforce diversity efforts has been our Diversity Supplements program. Through the Research Supplements to Promote Diversity in Health-Related Research program, investigators can apply for supplements to existing grants to support the involvement of researchers from diverse backgrounds, including those from underrepresented groups, in their research project. A similar supplement program, Research Supplements to Promote Re-Entry and Re-integration into Health-Related Research Careers, aims to support those individuals with a doctoral degree who have temporarily left the scientific workforce for reasons like childcare or eldercare and wish to return to research. The recently added Re-integration component of this program provides an opportunity for individuals at a range of research training and career levels, who are adversely affected by unsafe or discriminatory environments resulting from unlawful harassment to rapidly transition into safer and more supportive research environments. Unsafe environments may include sexual and gender harassment, harassment based on being a member of a racial, ethnic, sexual, or gender minority group, or other similar circumstances.

Although some progress has been made in increasing diversity at earlier career stages, individuals from underrepresented groups are still less likely to be hired into positions as independently funded faculty researchers. In response to this challenge, the NIH Common Fund recently introduced the Faculty Institutional Recruitment for Sustainable Transformation (FIRST) Program.[21] This unique program provides support to institutions to recruit diverse groups or "cohorts" of early-stage research faculty with the aim of transforming culture at NIH-funded extramural institutions by building a self-reinforcing community of scientists committed to diversity and inclusive excellence. The inaugural FIRST cohort was awarded and announced in the fall of 2021.

We acknowledge that although efforts to date have helped, they still fall short, and much more work remains to be done. NIMH plans to evaluate the effectiveness of its ongoing efforts and work with NIH-wide efforts and other stakeholders to identify gaps and opportunities for improvement. More importantly, NIMH considers these research training and career promotion programs as one tactic in an arsenal of approaches for addressing workforce diversity.

SUPPORTING RESEARCH ON MENTAL HEALTH DISPARITIES

Another factor contributing to the lack of diversity in the mental health research workforce has been the disconnect between mainstream research priorities and the interests of many scientists from racial and ethnic groups negatively impacted by health disparities. This mismatch was frequently mentioned in listening sessions conducted by the NIMH with BIPOC scientists in the spring and summer of 2021. We heard often of the frustration experienced by many when their scientific goals and interests were met with a lack of enthusiasm by peer reviewers and NIMH program officials. This mismatch makes it difficult for scientists from racial and ethnic minority groups to see paths to success in mental health research and contributes to the disparities seen in funding rates.[16,17] NIMH is reconfirming its commitment to research in health disparities, one area in particular that draws the scientific interests of many scientists from racial and ethnic minority groups. Over the past year, NIMH has conducted a series of webinars and workshops on minority mental health and mental health disparities and released a Request for Information seeking input from the broader community. These efforts led to the specification of a set of research priorities that focuses on community-based research, mechanistic-based approaches to understanding factors contributing to disparities, and targeted interventions aimed at these mechanisms to mitigate the disparities.[22] Building on these plans, NIMH will work toward sustained growth in the mental health disparities research portfolio through targeted Funding Opportunity Announcements, concerted outreach, and proactive engagement with researchers in the extramural community.

Fundamentally, the mismatch between mainstream priorities and the interests of BIPOC scientists is a product of systemic racism. Reviewers, program staff, and scientific leadership derive predominantly from an established majority culture, and the priorities articulated by NIMH and implemented by reviewers derive from those of the majority culture. In the absence of intentional actions to diversify our workforce, the homogeneity of this perspective (like culture more broadly) is self-perpetuating and will be resistant to change. Effectively identifying and addressing systemic racism and dismantling its impact on science will require both short- and long-term solutions.

Above, we discussed strategies being implemented to promote equity in funding decisions along with data suggesting that they are having a positive, near-term impact.

Another strategy to diversify the workforce is to change the culture within NIMH and NIH. To build a scientific leadership system that equitably reflects the priorities of all Americans, we need to recruit and build an Institute whose staff and leadership reflect the diversity of America. Efforts to do just that are underway. At the NIH level, the UNITE Initiative has been working to set NIH-wide strategies for equity, diversity, and inclusion.[23] Within NIMH, our own Anti-Racism Task Force has articulated a set of recommendations, centering on a transparent, data-driven approach to accountability. Both efforts emphasize a need for leadership across the Institute to listen to employees of color and other underrepresented groups; address hiring, promotion, and retention practices; require equity in opportunities for training and career development; and instill a culture of respect and inclusion that strives to eliminate race-based harassment and microaggressions. Although we hope these efforts will lead to lasting change within NIMH, we also hope to foster and support similar efforts in the wider mental health research community.

SUMMARY

It is clear to many in the mental health research community, and to the staff and leadership at NIMH, that the time to recommit to creating and sustaining an equitable, diverse, and inclusive workforce is now. This moment in time, marked by the coincident shocks of the COVID-19 pandemic and the escalation of police violence against people of color, is a watershed moment. Taking advantage of the increased focus on mental health in the context of these shocks, and the recognition that systemic racism has been hampering research that could be helping address the broader needs of individuals with mental illnesses, as well as their families and communities, is a moral and scientific imperative. Diversity is necessary for excellent science, and the cause of excellent science demands that we continue to identify and understand the structural obstacles to a diverse workforce, how they exert their effects, and how we can intentionally intervene to dismantle them. Here we have described the problem, and initial NIMH efforts to pave a way forward, including ensuring a just and equitable funding process, building a diverse workforce through training, and supporting research on health disparities. Recognizing that what we have done so far is not enough, we need to continue to search for innovative ways to improve and grow a diverse workforce, to establish their efficacy, and to implement those innovations wherever feasible. We cannot be distracted by efforts to defend the status quo, but instead must work to change established structural elements that impede progress toward equitable access to high-quality, evidence-based mental health care, and that starts with building an equitable and diverse mental health research workforce.

ACKNOWLEDGMENTS

The authors thank Ishmael Amarreh, PhD, Elan Cohen, MS, Dawn Morales, PhD, Uma Vaidyanathan, PhD, and Abera Wouhib, PhD for the analyses of funding rates by race described above and depicted in **Fig. 1**.

DISCLOSURE

The authors declare no commercial or financial conflicts of interest.

REFERENCES

1. McKnight-Eily LR, Okoro CA, Strine TW, et al. Racial and ethnic disparities in the prevalence of stress and worry, mental health conditions, and increased substance use among adults during the COVID-19 pandemic — United States, April and May 2020. MMWR Morb Mortal Wkly Rep 2021;70:162–6.

2. Stewart AJ. Dismantling structural racism in academic psychiatry to achieve workforce diversity. Am J Psychiatry 2021;178:224–8.

3. Swartz TH, Palermo AS, Masur SK, et al. The science and value of diversity: closing the gaps in our understanding of inclusion and diversity. J Infect Dis 2019; 220:S33–41.

4. Valantine HA, Collins FS. National Institutes of Health addresses the science of diversity. Proc Natl Acad Sci U S A 2015;112:12240–2.

5. American Psychiatric Association. Position statement on diversity and inclusion in the physician workforce. 2019. Available at: https://www.psychiatry.org/File% 20Library/About-APA/Organization-Documents-Policies/Policies/Position-Diversity-and-Inclusion-in-the-Physician-Workforce.pdf. Accessed November 6, 2021.

6. Moreno FA, Chhatwal J. Diversity and inclusion in psychiatry: the pursuit of health equity. Focus (Am Psychiatr Publ) 2020;18(1):2–7.

7. NIH Advisory Committee to the Director Working Group on Diversity. Racism in science report. 2021. Available at: https://acd.od.nih.gov/documents/presentations/02262021DiversityReport.pdf. Accessed October 31, 2021.

8. American Psychiatric Association. APA's apology to black, indigenous and people of color for its support of structural racism in psychiatry. 2021. Available at: https://www.psychiatry.org/newsroom/apa-apology-for-its-support-of-structural-racism-in-psychiatry. Accessed October 31, 2021.

9. American Psychiatric Association. Historical addendum to APA's apology to black, indigenous and people of color for its support of structural racism in psychiatry. 2021. Available at: https://www.psychiatry.org/newsroom/historical-addendum-to-apa-apology. Accessed October 31, 2021.

10. Collins FC. NIH stands against structural racism in biomedical research. 2021. Available at: https://www.nih.gov/about-nih/who-we-are/nih-director/statements/nih-stands-against-structural-racism-biomedical-research. Accessed October 31, 2021.

11. Gordon JA. NIMH director's statement on racism. 2020. Available at: https://www.nimh.nih.gov/news/science-news/2020/nimh-directors-statement-on-racism. Accessed October 31, 2021.

12. Fang D, Moy E, Colburn L, et al. Racial and ethnic disparities in faculty promotion in academic medicine. JAMA 2000;284:1085–92.

13. Stevens KR, Masters KS, Imoukhuede PI, et al. Fund black scientists. Cell 2021; 184:561–5.

14. Ginther DK, Schaffer WT, Schnell J, et al. Race, ethnicity, and NIH research awards. Science 2011;333(6045):1015–9.

15. Erosheva EA, Grant S, Chen M, et al. NIH peer review: criterion scores completely account for racial disparities in overall impact scores. Sci Adv 2020;6(23): eaaz4868.

16. Hoppe TA, Litovitz A, Willis KA, et al. Topic choice contributes to the lower rate of NIH awards to African-American/black scientists. Sci Adv 2019;5(10):eaaw7238.

17. Lauer MS, Doyle J, Wang J, et al. Associations of topic-specific peer review outcomes and institute and center award rates with funding disparities at the National Institutes of Health. Elife 2021;10:e67173.
18. Nakamura R, Mann LS, Lindner MD, et al. An experimental test of the effects of redacting grant applicant identifiers on peer review outcomes. eLife 2021;10: e71368.
19. Gordon JA. Steps toward equity at NIMH: an update. Available at: https://www.nimh.nih.gov/about/director/messages/2022/steps-toward-equity-at-nimh-an-update, 2022. Accessed March 28, 2022.
20. NIH BRAIN Initiative. Plan for enhancing diverse perspectives (PEDP). 2021. Available at: https://braininitiative.nih.gov/about/plan-enhancing-diverse-perspectives-pedp. Accessed October 31, 2021.
21. National Institutes of Health. Faculty institutional recruitment for sustainable transformation. 2021. Available at: https://commonfund.nih.gov/first. Accessed November 1, 2021.
22. National Institute of Mental Health. NIMH's approach to mental health disparities. 2021. Available at: https://www.nimh.nih.gov/about/organization/od/odwd/nimhs-approach-to-mental-health-disparities-research. Accessed November 1, 2021.
23. Collins FS, Adams AB, Aklin C, et al. Affirming NIH's commitment to addressing structural racism in the biomedical research enterprise. Cell 2021;184(12): 3075–9.

Telebehavioral Health
Workforce, Access, and Future Implications

Jennifer B. Reese, PsyD[a], Ujjwal Ramtekkar, MD, MBA, MPE[b],*

KEYWORDS

- Telehealth • Telebehavioral • Telepsychiatry • Psychiatry • Psychology
- Behavioral health

KEY POINTS

- Telebehavioral health (TBH) holds a great deal of promise in decreasing barriers to accessing care
- The success of TBH and Telehealth overall will depend on improvements in broadband access and infrastructure
- TBH has a unique appeal for the workforce in balancing work and home life
- Staff education in TBH delivery should be 2-fold in focus: (1) functionality and (2) translation of clinical skill and process to the virtual environment

INTRODUCTION

The use of telehealth for behavioral health services has been referred to as telepsychiatry, telepsychology, and telebehavioral health. As professionals from a variety of disciplines deliver behavioral health services (eg, Social Workers, Clinical Counselors, Psychologists, Psychiatrists, and so forth), in the interest of being inclusive in this article we will refer to telehealth as delivered in the context of behavioral health as telebehavioral health (TBH).

A growing body of literature substantiates TBH as an effective mode of service delivery for children, adolescents, and their families. Even before the coronavirus disease (COVID-19) pandemic, studies had established that TBH is feasible, well accepted and the interventions generated outcomes comparable to those delivered via in-person treatment.[1] Based on the mounting evidence of diagnostic validity and effectiveness of TBH across different disorders in children and adolescents, it has been recognized as a distinct venue instead of another modality to deliver care. Despite

This article originally appeared in *Psychiatric Clinics*, Volume 45 Issue 2, June 2022.
^a Department of Psychiatry and Behavioral Health, Nationwide Children's Hospital, 700 Children's Drive, Columbus, OH 43205, USA; ^b Department of Psychiatry, University of Missouri School of Medicine, 3 Hospital Drive, Columbia, MO, USA
* Corresponding author.
E-mail address: ramtekkaru@umsystem.edu

Child Adolesc Psychiatric Clin N Am 33 (2024) 87–93
https://doi.org/10.1016/j.chc.2023.06.010
1056-4993/24/© 2023 Elsevier Inc. All rights reserved.

childpsych.theclinics.com

the evidence, adoption of TBH was stagnated due to several factors including regulatory barriers posed by federal and state guidelines, lack of parity or even coverage of TBH services for reimbursement by payers, challenges with licensure requirement to use TBH across state lines, costs associated with technology, lack of interoperability and integration between telehealth platforms with common electronic medical records (EMR), availability of broadband Internet connectivity in the nonmetro and rural areas, and often lack of clear metrics of success or incentives for health care organizations and providers to embrace TBH as part of their care model.[2] Fortunately, the relaxation of regulations and coverage of TBH by insurance providers during the public health emergency in response to pandemic provided an opportunity for telehealth service delivery volume and applications across all levels of acuity to grow exponentially in ways that were previously unimagined.[3] The innovation and expansion TBH in the context of the pandemic will surely generate additional literature evaluating its efficacy and outcomes. In this article, we provide an overview of TBH implications as well as our experience at a large pediatric behavioral health institution in the context of quadruple aim for health care with focus on provider and patient experience, workforce, access to care, and future direction for newer models of care.

Equity and Access to Telebehavioral Health

The need for TBH adoption highlighted the existing disparities in equitable access to resources. Historically, the access to broadband has been lower for rural populations. In addition, there is a significant gap in access and adoption of technology by race (16% in Black individuals vs 79% in White individuals).[4] Telehealth and transition to virtual learning by schools laid bare the lagging infrastructure of our telecommunications grids.[2,5] Some families simply had no access to reliable broadband connections, resulting in their care occurring largely via telephone. Language barriers also came into focus, as many telehealth platforms and supporting documentation were initially available only in English.

On the positive side, for rural communities, seeking mental health services has historically been curtailed due to concerns around stigma and privacy, as well as geographic isolation and transportation challenges. TBH can eliminate all of these barriers. Even beyond rural communities, TBH was an equalizer for families who struggled with access to reliable transportation or for families with multiple young children who would either need to attend the appointment with the identified patient or for whom childcare would otherwise have to be arranged. These barriers were easily removed by their ability to log on for their TBH session from right within their home or community. The positive benefit of telehealth services with families whose primary language was not English was that our interpretation services previously relied heavily upon interpreters attending sessions in person within the clinic, whereas with telehealth they could join these sessions virtually, in an on-demand fashion. Lastly, the need for digital literacy in addition to health literacy seems to be important as TBH becomes an integral part of care delivery in rural and underserved populations.

Equity and Diversity in the Workforce

TBH provides benefits for the workforce as well. Individual practitioners in rural communities may be able to expand their catchment areas by minimizing or eliminating the need for families to attend sessions in person, thereby removing physical distance as a barrier. Virtual platforms also allow rural practitioners and their patients greater, more convenient access to specialists who may not be conveniently located. Rather than having to commute to work in an urban center to earn competitive wages, these clinicians can remain in the communities in which they reside.

For the practitioners themselves, being able to deliver services via TBH can allow them greater flexibility in their work day, particularly if they are able to deliver these services from home. This can be particularly attractive for those with caregiver responsibilities for their own children or other family members, as they can be more accessible as needs arise. Being able to work remotely also allows for greater freedom of choice in terms of whereby one resides, thereby addressing the economic burden posed by moving to urban areas. Anecdotally, clinicians have indicated that working from home makes it easier for them to offer evening appointments, which are typically in high demand by patient families.

Telebehavioral Health Models for Workforce Development

A critical shortage of trained behavioral health providers is well established. The gap between demand for services and supply of providers continues to be a challenge to support the current needs for youth mental health. For example, despite the 22% growth in the number of child and adolescent psychiatrists (CAPs) over the past decade, it still leaves more than 70% of counties in the United States without any CAPs[6] and more than 50% of youth without any services. As a result, relying on the traditional models of care is not sustainable and exploring ways to develop alternative means of meeting behavioral health care needs, such as through primary care providers (PCPs) and school health resources is imperative. PCPs are often the front line for pediatric patients presenting with behavioral health concerns but can experience some hesitance in initiating pharmacologic interventions that are less familiar to them. Telehealth-based models such as Project ECHO, Child Psychiatry Access Projects (CPAPs), and crisis consultations have been well-positioned to maximize the expertise of specialists to reach the communities through their primary care medical homes and school health clinics.

We adapted the established model of Project Extension for Community Healthcare Outcomes (Project ECHO) for the capacity development of our primary care workforce in the management of common behavioral health presentations of youth.[7] Project ECHO uses a cohort-based teleconsultation model whereby a multidisciplinary "hub" team of specialists facilitates learning and shares expertise to the "spokes" of community providers over a videoconferencing platform. Project ECHO involves short "evidence-based didactics" wherein hub team members lead brief presentations to build content knowledge followed by case-based learning whereby the participants present real-world cases. In presenting cases, the participants are able to get live consultation from their peers and experts on the hub team to improve their comfort and competence. We demonstrated self-reported improvement in overall capacity, comfort, and competence as well as objective practice change based on insurance claims data for the providers participating in our cohorts.[6] We have trained more than 100 pediatric practices more than 37 rural counties in the state who serve as the first access point for noncrisis behavioral health concerns for youth.

Similarly, we have been able to use virtual platforms for other types of provider-to-provider consultation specially for PCPs who have completed training through Project ECHO. Building on the existing CPAP model which is largely phone based, we incorporated the use of scheduled video consultation for PCPs.[8] Our program allowed scheduling a video appointment with a psychiatrist within a day to provide individualized case consultation or more general treatment guidance. In addition, the case manager provides linkage and referral support within the community so that the PCP can confidently refer and implement the treatment plan discussed during the call. The service allows the youth and families to access services within their primary care medical home and behavioral health agencies without leaving their communities. The telehealth-based, provider-to-provider consultation model not only mitigated the crisis of long wait times for specialty care but also created the capacity for the specialists to see youth with complex behavioral health needs. Our preliminary data indicate that the primary reason for calls is for medication management or referrals but the recommendations after case discussion are more likely to be therapy interventions and local resources thus reinforcing the evidence-based treatment modalities with judicious use of medications and avoidance of polypharmacy.

We have also realized the benefits of the virtual landscape for collaboration and consultation in crisis. Crisis clinicians are now able to consult with emergency department providers in surrounding areas to determine if a patient truly needs to make the journey to our psychiatric crisis department, or if with some safety planning and other support identification they can return home with caregivers. Along with saving these families a drive to another location, this also saves them the wait time, the strain of sharing their story with a new set of providers, and additional health care costs.

Workforce Education and Training for Telebehavioral Health

Training to adapt clinical functions to telebehavioral health

Our large pediatric behavioral health department learned important lessons in the rapid adoption of telehealth services[2] First and foremost was the translation of our suicide screening and risk assessment protocols designed for clinic visits to the virtual realm. Information that could be taken for granted in a clinic environment (eg, location of patient, available adults) were unknown unless intentionally gathered in the session. We established a protocol by which providers and clinicians first established the location of the patient and others available to provide support in that environment should a crisis arise. By routinely gathering that information at the outset, providers could then focus on assessment and providing support as urgent needs arose rather than having to pause and gather this information, or worse yet, not having it in the event the telehealth session was disconnected for some reason. We educated our staff on this adaptation of our suicide prevention protocols through a detailed document outlining these changes, as well as a visual workflow document. As other resources were developed nationally we integrated those guidelines into materials available to our staff.

Educating staff on TBH practice would be a substantial undertaking even in ordinary times. Attempting to do so in the context of the COVID-19 pandemic and societal tension of the past year proved to be incredibly challenging. Stress and learning literature indicate that stress can enhance learning and memory when experienced in the context of the learning event, but the events of the past year were more chronic and pervasive in nature, likely leading to impaired cognitive performance and memory.[9,10] Therefore, we determined that the best course of action was to focus on the functionality of performing TBH(eg, Initiating virtual sessions through our EMR, documentation requirements, troubleshooting with families experiencing difficulty accessing their virtual visit, and so forth), emphasizing that their prepandemic clinical skills were still applicable. As mentioned previously, pressing safety considerations associated with suicide screening and risk assessment and relevant adaptations were also educated. Additionally, we created telehealth support office hours where staff could join a Zoom session on designated days and times to talk with internal experts for advice, problem solving, and troubleshooting.

Training to develop competencies for effective telebehavioral health

Once our staff had roughly 90 days of experience with delivering TBH services, we generated additional education content to further develop their skills. These consisted of a series of on-demand learning modules covering such topics as session engagement strategies, using motivational interviewing in the context of telebehavioral health and addressing and managing safety concerns (**Table 1**). We obtained continuing education (CE) credit for these modules, as many other CE events were either canceled or postponed, leading to difficulty in accumulating hours for licensure renewal.

Like many institutions, our organization historically outgrew space more quickly than we could build it, but remote work and telehealth both offered solutions to these problems not previously considered. Furthermore, our staff have only experienced the utilization of telehealth under remote working conditions, so we have had to be mindful of separating the 2 concepts (ie, telehealth does not equal working remotely). As we prepare for life in postpandemic times, discussions have turned to how and when telehealth should be used for services. Factors requiring consideration include practitioner skill and preference, patient/family preference and resources, and defining what patients are or are not a good fit for telehealth (eg, those experiencing chronic, acute safety concerns are not a good fit for telehealth). We are in the process of developing decision trees which first outline establishing whether the patient/family has the resources necessary (eg, reliable broadband network access; technological devices such as smartphones, tablets, or computers; comfort and confidence in using digital devices) to engage in telehealth services. Should they have these necessary resources, the next step in the decision tree will be establishing whether the patient and/or caregiver has any contraindicating factors for engaging in telehealth services, which would likely lead to poorer outcomes as compared with in-person care. Lastly, if both telehealth and in-person options are left on the table, patient/family preference will be considered.

Patient Satisfaction

The rapid adoption and continued utilization of TBH by providers as well as patients likely indicated acceptance and satisfaction with the services provided. Patient satisfaction surveys conducted at our organization beginning in August 2020 indicated that

Table 1
Patient satisfaction survey data from 2650 unique Behavioral Health patients from 8/1/2020 to 9/28/2020

Experience Rating	Strongly Agree (%)	Agree (%)	Somewhat Agree (%)	Disagree (%)	Strongly Disagree (%)
Telehealth improves my access to health care services.	65.36	23.09	8.38	2.15	1.02
My overall experience with NCH telehealth was good.	73.58	21.81	2.91	1.09	0.60
If given the option, I would use video visit for future appointments.	52.91	21.13	16.75	6.79	2.42

Experience Rating	Better (%)	Equal (%)	Worse (%)	Not Sure (%)
Compared with the level of care received during an in-person visit, the level of care received during the telemedicine appointment was…	11.21	64.72	4.79	7.36

the vast majority of parents and caregivers experienced the level of care they received via telehealth as being equal to or better than the care they had received in person (**Box 1**). That trend has held in subsequent surveys. Patient families also indicated believing that telehealth improved their access to health care (88.45% agreed or strongly agreed this was the case). If given the choice, just less than 75% agreed or strongly agreed that they would continue to use video visits for future health care appointments. Just more than 95% indicated that they had a good overall experience with telehealth in our system. Some of the qualitative responses indicated that when the telemedicine appointment experience was rated as worse, it was largely attributed to the technical or technological difficulties during the initiation of the telehealth visit, not related to the clinical experience. Several youth using TBH indicated that they were hesitant in visiting with the behavioral health professional for years due to stigma, perceived impressions about the psychiatry or therapy clinics, and/ or discomfort and anxiety around talking about sensitive and often emotionally overwhelming topics. However, they only agreed to engage in initial evaluation visits due to the availability of TBH which provided a sense of psychological safety as they were in their familiar or home environment, and it mimicked their most common mode of social communication which is audiovisual via smartphones, tablets, or computers.

Future Directions

As we enter the "new normal" of health care, the experiences during the pandemic will make TBH an integral part of care delivery as a solution to improve equity and access to diverse populations irrespective of their geographic location and socioeconomic status. To optimally use TBH, it is crucial to break the traditional dichotomy of in person versus TBH care. The true value is in the "hybrid model" of using both in person and TBH during the episode of care based on the clinical acuity, interventions, patient factors, and clinician factors. Although, the continued progress is possible only if the regulatory changes are continued and made permanent to allow services and remove barriers that mandate the in-person visits to initiate care. In addition, active investment in the infrastructure for broadband and connectivity is imperative to further bridge the chasm and disparities between urban and rural communities. Furthermore, creative solutions like creating access points at schools, libraries, or local clinics could address the barriers related to social determinants of health. In the interim—phone only visits for limited use cases could continue to be of value for many individuals.

TBH has demonstrated the opportunities to recruit and retain a diverse workforce without the need to leave their communities. It is imperative that the health systems, academic centers, and state regulations allow the design of remote work models for clinicians to work in the local hubs to provide culturally sensitive care customized to the needs of their respective communities. However, there should be emphasis on recognizing that TBH is a distinct venue and modality that requires training to acquire unique competencies to deliver effective and authentic care. The different disciplines within behavioral health would benefit from replicating the efforts by the American

---

Box 1
Education modules developed.

The Basics of Telebehavioral Health

Addressing & Managing Safety Concerns

Using Motivational Interviewing to Improve Telebehavioral Health Practice

Academy of Child and Adolescent Psychiatry to implement a national telepsychiatry curriculum.[6]

DISCLOSURE

The authors have nothing to disclose.

REFERENCES

1. Academy of Child A. Psychiatry Committee on Telepsychiatry, A., & Committee on Quality Issues, A). AACAP OFFICIAL ACTION Clinical Update: Telepsychiatry With Children and Adolescents American Academy of Child and Adolescent Psychiatry (AACAP) Committee on Telepsychiatry and AACAP Committee on Quality Issues. J Am Acad Child Adolesc Psychiatry 2017. https://doi.org/10.1016/j.jaac.2017.07.008.
2. Ramtekkar U, Bridge JA, Thomas G, et al. Pediatric telebehavioral health: A transformational shift in care delivery in the era of COVID-19. JMIR Ment Health 2020;7(Issue 9). https://doi.org/10.2196/20157.
3. CDC. Using Telehealth to Expand Access to Essential Health Services during the COVID-19 Pandemic. Centers Dis Control Prev 2020.
4. Walker DM, Hefner JL, Fareed N, et al. Exploring the digital divide: Age and race disparities in use of an inpatient portal. Telemed E-Health 2020;26(5). https://doi.org/10.1089/tmj.2019.0065.
5. Ekezue BF, Bushelle-Edghill J, Dong S, et al. The effect of broadband access on electronic patient engagement activities: Assessment of urban-rural differences. J Rural Health 2021. https://doi.org/10.1111/jrh.12598.
6. Hostutler CA, Valleru J, Maciejewski HM, et al. Improving Pediatrician's Behavioral Health Competencies Through the Project ECHO Teleconsultation Model. Clin Pediatr 2020. https://doi.org/10.1177/0009922820927018.
7. Hager B, Hasselberg M, Arzubi E, et al. Leveraging behavioral health expertise: Practices and potential of the project ECHO approach to virtually integrating care in underserved areas. Psychiatr Serv 2018;69(4). https://doi.org/10.1176/appi.ps.201700211.
8. Sarvet B, Gold J, Bostic JQ, et al. Improving access to mental health care for children: The Massachusetts Child Psychiatry Access Project. Pediatrics 2010. https://doi.org/10.1542/peds.2009-1340.
9. Joëls M, Pu Z, Wiegert O, et al. Learning under stress: how does it work? Trends Cogn Sci 2006;10(4). https://doi.org/10.1016/j.tics.2006.02.002.
10. Smeets T, Giesbrecht T, Jelicic M, et al. Context-dependent enhancement of declarative memory performance following acute psychosocial stress. Biol Psychol 2007;76(1–2). https://doi.org/10.1016/j.biopsycho.2007.07.001.

AACAP's Strategic Plans to Enhance the Diversity of the Child Psychiatry and Child Mental Health Workforce Across all Mission Areas

Tashalee R. Brown, MD, PhD[a],*, Tami D. Benton, MD[b], Warren Yiu Kee Ng, MD, MPH[c,d]

KEYWORDS

- Diversity • Equity • Inclusion • Mental health • Physician workforce

KEY POINTS

- Promoting diversity, equity, and inclusion (DEI) goals across American Academy of Child and Adolescent Psychiatry's mission areas required embedding DEI initiatives into the organization on a structural level.
- Support for a pipeline of child and adolescent psychiatrists involved enhancing leadership opportunities, expansion of mentorship, and promoting diversity in scholarly activities.
- Monitoring DEI activities at an organizational level is important to sustain progress toward goals.

INTRODUCTION

The mission of the American Academy of Child and Adolescent Psychiatry (AACAP) is to promote the healthy development of children, adolescents, and families through advocacy, education, and research and to meet the professional needs of child and adolescent psychiatrists throughout their careers. In order to accomplish this goal, the organization has prioritized the importance of diversity, equity, and inclusion (DEI). In order to have transformational influence and to create change, the support and alignment of organizational leadership is a critical and key component of the

[a] David Geffen School of Medicine, University of California Los Angeles, Los Angeles, CA, USA; [b] Department of Child and Adolescent Psychiatry and Behavioral Sciences, Children's Hospital of Philadelphia, HUB – Center for Clinical Collaboration, 3501 Civic Center Boulevard, 12th Floor, Philadelphia, PA 19104, USA; [c] Columbia University Irving Medical Center, New York-Presbyterian Hospital, 3959 Broadway, MSCH 6 North, New York, NY 10032, USA; [d] Columbia University Irving Medical Center, Morgan Stanley Children's Hospital, New York, USA
* Corresponding author. UCLA Psychiatry House Staff Office, 760 Westwood Plaza, Suite B7-357, Los Angeles, CA 90024.
E-mail address: TashaleeBrown@mednet.ucla.edu

Child Adolesc Psychiatric Clin N Am 33 (2024) 95–109
https://doi.org/10.1016/j.chc.2023.09.002
1056-4993/24/© 2023 Elsevier Inc. All rights reserved.

strategy. AACAP's President and the CEO/Executive Director, Heidi Fordi, work synergistically to achieve the DEI goals with members and staff. This article will discuss AACAP's strategic plan for transforming how the organization can expand and amplify the richness of diversity within the field of child and adolescent psychiatry. Key aspects of achieving this goal are diversifying the physician workforce and increasing representation in AACAP's membership and leadership. Three main areas will be discussed in this article: promoting DEI across all mission areas, creating a pipeline of child and adolescent psychiatrists, and monitoring DEI activities and progress on an organizational level. Lists of key points related to each of these areas will be expanded and articulated with examples.

These DEI initiatives are consistent with workforce diversity efforts by the Association of American Medical Colleges (AAMC), American Association of Directors of Psychiatric Residency Training (AADPRT), Association of Directors of Medical Student Education in Psychiatry, and the American Psychiatric Association. For example, AADPRT established a Diversity and Inclusion Committee, which systematically investigated diversity among psychiatry program directors throughout the United States and Canada.[1] Similarly, the AAMC released a 10-part strategic plan, which included an action plan to increase the number of diverse medical school applicants and matriculants.[2] AACAP's leadership reviewed these efforts in arriving at the strategy to move these priorities forward.

BACKGROUND

Nonviolent direct action seeks to create such a crisis and establish such creative tension that a community that has constantly refused to negotiate is forced to confront the issue. It seeks to dramatize the issue that it can no longer be ignored.
– Martin Luther King Jr.

The current mental health-care workforce does not match the current patient population of children, adolescents, and families most in need of mental health services. Unfortunately, Black, Indigenous, People of Color (BIPOC) individuals and other marginalized, minoritized, and underserved individuals lack representation in the existing mental health-care workforce.[3,4] The benefits of having a more diverse workforce are shown through existing evidence that provider–patient concordance in cultural backgrounds result in more positive perceptions of care and better rates of adherence to treatment.[5] Some studies have identified improved health outcomes when there is a health-care provider who represents the community served.[5,6] Furthermore, marginalized and minoritized communities experience more barriers to care, which are rooted in social determinants of health.[7] There is also increasing recognition that racism is an important social determinant of health, especially for children and adolescents.[8] For instance, provider level implicit bias is implicated in racial/ethnic disparities in mental health outcomes,[9] a risk that may be mitigated by diversifying the workforce. The importance of transforming the diversity of the workforce in addition to transforming the workplace itself are amplified in the work of Dr Camara Phyllis Jones, where she presents a theoretic framework for understanding racism on 3 levels: personally mediated, internalized, and institutionalized (**Table 1**).[10,11]

There is a long history of barriers to workforce diversity within medicine and health care. Gross inequities exist all along the pipeline to becoming a physician, starting at elementary school within your community. Over the years, very deliberate efforts to impede diversification of the workforce have occurred, such as the shutting down of historically Black medical colleges in the wake of the Flexner report. This resulted in drastic decreases in the number of Black physicians within the field of medicine.[12,13]

Table 1
A theoretic framework for understanding racism on 3 levels: personally mediated, internalized, and institutionalized[11]

Levels of Racism	Definition
Personally mediated	It is defined as, "prejudice and discrimination, where prejudice means differential assumptions about the abilities, motives, and intentions of others according to their race, and discrimination means differential actions toward others according to their race."
Internalized	It is defined as, "acceptance by members of the stigmatized races of negative messages about their own abilities and intrinsic worth. It is characterized by their not believing in others who look like them, and not believing in themselves. It involves accepting limitations to one's own full humanity, including one's spectrum of dreams, one's right to self-determination, and one's range of allowable self-expression."
Institutionalized	It is defined as, "differential access to the goods, services, and opportunities of society by race. Institutionalized racism is normative, sometimes legalized, and often manifests as inherited disadvantage. It is structural, having been codified in our institutions of custom, practice, and law, so there need not be an identifiable perpetrator."

Such structural issues result in what is often referred to as the "leaky pipeline." This is when organizations attract BIPOC scholars but their numbers diminish over time due to structural barriers such as the lack of, or poor quality of, mentorship and support. This results in devaluation (ie, minimizing ambitions), underrepresentation of BIPOC scholars in leadership roles, and gatekeeping practices, including lack of transparency in hiring and promotions.[14,15] Acknowledging the history of racism and other forms of oppression within medicine is an important first step toward directly addressing and dismantling systemic and structural barriers to diversity.

These barriers to workforce diversity have disproportionally influenced the child and adolescent psychiatry workforce resulting in disparities in care for minoritized youth in our country. Given that minoritized providers treat a larger proportion of ethnic and racially minoritized patients than White providers[6] and the shifting demographics of children and adolescents in the United States toward increasing diversity identified in the 2019 US census report[16] supports the urgent need for diversifying the workforce in child and adolescent psychiatry.

Understanding the current data available on diversity in medicine, and specifically child and adolescent psychiatry, helps to inform ongoing challenges and opportunities. In reviewing the AAMC Diversity in Medicine Facts and Figures 2019, one can see the applicant, matriculant, and graduate data from the academic year 2018 to 2019.[17] First, one important finding from this data is that race and ethnicity data are missing for 13.7% active physicians overall.[17] Second, there seems to be greater diversity among medical students and those entering child and adolescent psychiatry residency compared with the practicing physicians in the field (**Table 2**). These findings suggest opportunities for growth concerning representation in child and adolescent psychiatry. However, we also see an increase in the total number of child and adolescent psychiatrists in recent years, which may facilitate efforts to diversify this workforce. For example, the total number of active physicians in child and adolescent psychiatry was 9966 in 2021.[18] From 2016 to 2021, there has been a 9.9% increase in the number of active physicians in child and adolescent psychiatry compared with 0.2% in psychiatry and 2.5% in pediatrics.[19] In regards to female gender representation among first-year ACGME child and adolescent psychiatry residents and fellows,

Table 2
The percentage of child and adolescent psychiatrists, child and adolescent psychiatry residents, and medical school matriculants who identify as certain racial/ethnic groups

Race/Ethnicity	AACAP Membership in 2023	Child and Adolescent Psychiatrists in 2021[33]	Child and Adolescent Psychiatry Resident in 2021[34]	Medical School Matriculants in 2021–2022[35]
Native Hawaiian/Pacific Islander	1.3%	0.1%	0.3%	0.4%
American Indian/Alaska native	0.4%	0.3%	1.3%	1.0%
Multiple race	-	1.6%	-	-
Black/African American	8.5%	7.9%	9.8%	11.3%
Hispanic	7.0%	8.3%	11.3%	12.7%
Asian	12.8%	21.8%	29%	26.5%
White	44.7%	50.9%	44%	51.5%
Other race	1.4%	0.9%	3.7%	3.9%
Missing/unknown	24.1%	8.3%	0.1%	3.5%

60.5% identified as women,[20] and there has been a 6.5% increase in overall numbers from 2016 to 2021.[21] This is in contrast to medical school matriculants in which AAMC data showed that 57% of applicants were women in 2022 to 2023.[22] Although this is encouraging, it still falls short of the representation needed to best serve the diverse children, adolescents, and families.

Recent Supreme Court rulings, which upended the use of affirmative action in college admissions, may also influence the pipeline for the recruitment of a diverse physician workforce in medical schools.[23,24] These Supreme court rulings can have an influence on the health outcomes of minoritized patients because it is known that Black people living in counties with more Black primary care physicians have lower mortality rates.[23] Furthermore, minoritized patients with providers from the same race or ethnic background reported greater satisfaction with their care.[23] Thus, efforts are needed more than ever to rectify the shortage of BIPOC individuals in the physician workforce.

PROMOTING DEI GOALS ACROSS AACAPs MISSION AREAS

AACAP was founded in 1953 and has targeted the needs of its membership during the decades. AACAP's Diversity and Culture Committee started in 1994 with the visionary leadership of Drs Jeanne Spurlock and Ian Canino. Over time, it has grown with the creation of initially the Black and Latino Caucuses in 2010, then the International Medical Graduates in 2012, and most recently, the Asian Caucus in 2018. A new emerging Arab Caucus is taking the next steps. These Caucuses reflect some of the largest BIPOC groups in AACAP's membership (see **Table 2**) and have been invaluable in creating a community of belonging, leadership opportunities, education, and advocacy. In the last 10 years, there has been trends toward increased leadership diversity with 4 women presidents, including AACAP's president-elect, Dr Tami D. Benton, there will be 9 women presidents (27%) and 2 Black/African American and 2 Asian (4 BIPOC, 12%).

In 2020, AACAP president Gabrielle Carlson appointed the inaugural Working Group to Promote Health Equity and Combat Racism led by Drs Melvin Oatis, Lisa M. Cullins, and Tami D. Benton, with Director Carmen J. Thornton. The Working Group collaborated closely with the AACAP's Diversity and Culture Committee, in partnership with

AACAP's Black, Latino, International Medical Graduate, and Asian Caucuses and leadership to help develop an action plan, which highlighted the initial 4 priority areas that needed more attention and effort to address the challenges of health inequities (**Fig. 1**). This included awareness, advocacy, workforce and professional development, and national partnerships and linkages.

The first priority area is increasing awareness on mental health disparities and promising practices via the AACAP website and other communication channels while consulting national experts to identify important clinical practice and research topics. The goal of these activities is to offer AACAP members and other mental health professionals' evidence-based solutions to improve health equity in clinical practice and research.

The second priority area is advocacy, which aims to engage key stakeholders and policymakers, at the state and local levels to improve health outcomes for BIPOC children and adolescents. The goals of these activities are to influence and develop policy recommendations and change to address disparities.

The third priority area is workforce and professional development, which aims to increase opportunities for professional development, diversity workforce recruitment, and research to address mental health inequities. AACAP's goals in this area are to promote workforce recruitment and mentorships and build a greater body of research addressing mental health disparities in BIPOC youth.

The fourth priority area is national partnership and linkages in which AACAP will to establish partnerships with other national professional medical associations, as well as federal partners promoting increased focus on disparities in BIPOC youth. AACAP's goal in this area is to support its peer associations in creating equity-focused policy statements and participate in meetings of national partners to enhance national efforts to address mental health-care disparities.

These 4 priority areas were supported and expanded by AACAP's president Warren Ng's presidential initiative CAPture Belonging. This presidential initiative made DEI and Belonging the highest level of priority. The Working Group thus became a presidential task force to advance the 4 target areas. With regard to awareness, this initiative

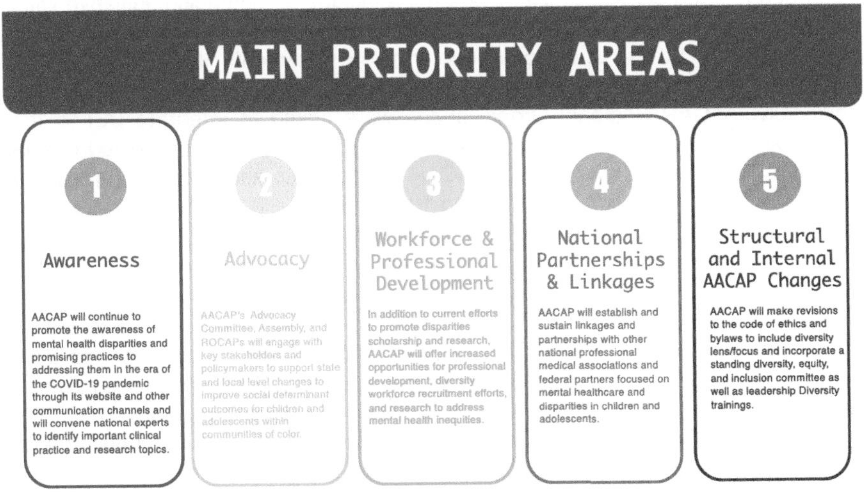

MAIN PRIORITY AREAS

1

Awareness

AACAP will continue to promote the awareness of mental health disparities and promising practices to addressing them in the era of the COVID-19 pandemic through its website and other communication channels and will convene national experts to identify important clinical practice and research topics.

2

Advocacy

AACAP's Advocacy Committee, Assembly, and ROCAP's will engage with key stakeholders and policymakers to support state and local level changes to improve social determinant outcomes for children and adolescents within communities of color.

3

Workforce & Professional Development

In addition to current efforts to promote disparities scholarship and research, AACAP will offer increased opportunities for professional development, diversity workforce recruitment efforts, and research to address mental health inequities.

4

National Partnerships & Linkages

AACAP will establish and sustain linkages and partnerships with other national professional medical associations and federal partners focused on mental healthcare and disparities in children and adolescents.

5

Structural and Internal AACAP Changes

AACAP will make revisions to the code of ethics and bylaws to include diversity lens/focus and incorporate a standing diversity, equity, and inclusion committee as well as leadership Diversity trainings.

Fig. 1. AACAP's comprehensive action plan to address mental health inequity among BIPOC children during the era of coronavirus disease 2019. AACAP's strategic plan identified main priority areas of awareness, advocacy, and workforce and professional development, national partnerships and linkages, and structural and internal AACAP changes.

produced several *AACAP News* articles, virtual fora, resource libraries focused on DEI,[25] lecture series, grants, and facts for families focusing on effects of racism on children.[26] Awareness was also enhanced with the Program Committee embracing presidential initiative in expanding and enhancing DEI content, presentations, and events at AACAP's Annual Meeting. There will also be an inaugural DEI reception acknowledging the contributions of the Caucuses and Diversity and Culture Committees and partnerships. Finally, the presidential initiative activated committees and members who were submitting presentations to be mindful of DEI content and health equity.

Highlighting advocacy efforts, the second priority, included increased efforts and projects with the Department of Governmental Affairs (DGA). This included the Advocacy Committee, Political Action Committee, Grassroots Advocacy Liaison program, and other lobbying activities. The DGA integrated a DEI lens in their priorities, with DEI-focused efforts during the legislative summit, and DEI-focused policy and organizational statements.

Importantly, workforce and professional development have been increasingly prioritized by the CAPture Belonging initiative. AACAP's committees and their leadership have received direct guidance to integrate greater diversity among the committee membership, adding DEI to their charge, and enhancing DEI within their areas of focus. The DEI Emerging Leaders fellowship program was instrumental in expanding the leadership opportunities for diverse trainees within strategic AACAP components such as the Council and *the Journal of the American Academy of Child and Adolescent Psychiatry (JAACAP)* originally. Creating additional DEI-specific continuing medical education activities and webinars, developing the diversity and culture and microaggressions curriculum, and developing the excellence through mentorship series were also established.

For the fourth priority area, national partnerships and linkage efforts were prioritized with organizations such as the Association of Minority Health Professions Schools, Student National Medical Association, The Latino Medical Student Association, and Association of Native American Medical Students.

Finally, the CAPture Belonging initiative developed a fifth priority area focusing on structural and internal AACAP changes. Efforts include an antiracism initiative within *JAACAP* as well as making changes in AACAP's governing documents such as the Bylaws, Code of Ethics, and Committee mission statements through the AACAP Council, the governing board of directors that approves all organizational priorities. Additionally, AACAP Regional Organizations were asked to integrate DEI to their work locally and reporting on their progress. An updated and standardized method of collecting of demographic data of AACAP membership and program participants throughout the organization was initiated to better understand the makeup of the AACAP community and measure change over time.

DEI EFFORTS TO SUPPORT A PIPELINE OF CHILD AND ADOLESCENT PSYCHIATRISTS

Creating and sustaining a pipeline for diverse child and adolescent psychiatrists is critical to AACAP and its DEI goals. The culture and the community of trainees and early career psychiatrists to help advance DEI issues and create belonging have been integral to this goal. AACAP's leadership has been supportive of continued investment in DEI efforts but has been particularly impressed with the initiatives of the Medical Student and Resident (MSR) Committee and Early Career Psychiatrist and Diversity and Culture Committees. They have been very intentional about developing strategies to increase diversity along all dimensions early on and collaborating with other components of AACAP synergistically.

Trainees, early career psychiatrists, and more senior members from diverse backgrounds actively participate in mentorship. Both the MSR Committee and the Diversity and Culture Committee and Caucuses have developed powerful and robust mentoring programs that support diverse individuals throughout the journey of training to becoming a child and adolescent psychiatrist.

AACAP has invested in several DEI initiatives to support a pipeline of child and adolescent psychiatrists. First, the Program Committee for AACAP's Annual Meeting, which is among the largest and most influential committees, has incorporated a DEI lens to all their submissions to ensure inclusivity of diverse scholars and perspectives. In addition, they have worked to obtain feedback from participants about DEI, which helps to shape the membership experience. They also instituted limits on the number of submissions any one individual can submit to create presentation opportunities for a wider group of individuals. Secondly, there is the AACAP's early pipeline workforce development mentorship and networking program designed to introduce minority and underrepresented undergraduate students to child and adolescent psychiatry as a career. This was spearheaded by Dr Lisa Cullins and Director Carmen Thornton in 2017. Undergraduate students at the junior and senior level are selected to participate in mentorship and academic programming to foster interest in child and adolescent psychiatry, thus building connections with mentors within the AACAP community. Another targeted initiative is the AACAP Diversity, Equity and Inclusion Emerging Leaders Fellowship started in 2021 to include Fellowships at the governing council and *JAACAP*. These opportunities offered leadership and mentorship experience within the Council and *JAACAP*.[27] These programs were expanded in 2022 to include the Program Committee and Department of Government Affairs. These key leadership opportunities provide a leadership role within AACAP structures to ensure the inclusion of diverse trainee voices and mentorship for leadership. Leadership opportunities had already existed in both the Council and *JAACAP* but these new Emerging Leadership opportunities increased the opportunities to involve diverse trainees early in their career to learn more about AACAP as an organization.

Third, AACAP's latest 2 Abramson grants were awarded to DEI-focused projects: Engaging a New Generation of Trainees: Amplifying Voices of Color (2022) and Child and Adolescent Psychiatry Diversity, Equity, and Inclusivity in Research Pipeline Initiative (2023). These 2 unique programs involved diverse member leaders as well as early career psychiatrists and trainees. The first project targets the recruitment of diverse trainees by having them see themselves represented by diverse members in videos about a career in child and adolescent psychiatry. This project was intended to be posted on the AACAP website and used to promote child and adolescent psychiatry to colleges, training programs, and communities.[28] This has inspired a NexGen mentorship taskforce that has created more opportunities to promote DEI priorities. The second grant is a program specifically to support and mentor diverse physician scientists within child and adolescent psychiatry. By creating a community of diverse researchers with educational and mentorship opportunities, they can gain insights and the wisdom of others. These 2 grants aim to increase the number, diversity, and representation of child and adolescent mental health researchers and clinicians.

MONITORING ORGANIZATIONAL LEVEL DEI ACTIVITIES AND PROGRESS TOWARD GOALS

Within AACAP, we have identified specific areas of further development for DEI initiatives, which include the *JAACAP journal family*, AACAP Committees, Program Committee and

Annual Meeting, AACAP Assembly of Regional Organizations, Membership, and the Department of Government Affairs.

Journal of the American Academy of Child and Adolescent Psychiatry Journal Family

The JAACAP leadership with Editor in Chief, Dr Douglas Novins and Associate Editor, Rob Althoff and Managing Director/Journal Department Director, of Mary Billingsley, shared their vision of An Antiracist Journal in 2020.[29] They pledged commitment to become a journal that is antiracist at every level and pledge to solicit and disseminate literature that addresses systemic racism and its effects on children, adolescents, and families. They appointed a new Assistant Editor for Health Equity and Antiracism, Dr Eraka Bath, and Deputy Editor for DEI, Dr Wanjiku Njoroge, and they articulated a call for articles on the effects of race, racism, social justice, and health equity in child and adolescent psychiatry. Another important part of this initiative is to make the *JAACAP* editorial board inclusive and representative of the community it serves by tracking self-reported sociodemographic information of its editorial board. As of 2022, Senior Editors (ie, Editor-in-Chief, Associate Editor, and Deputy Editors, n = 10) includes 4 men (40%), 6 women (60%), 1 Asian (1%), 1 Black/African American (1%), and 8 White (80%).[30] Thus, BIPOC representation at the highest level of the editorial board remains a challenge. They have updated the editorial process to incorporate consideration of diversity within all articles under review and revised recruitment efforts to make the journal mastheads more inclusive. These efforts are in line with National Institute of Health recognition of the need to promote diversity among scholars.[31] These efforts and others aim to create opportunities for BIPOC authors in the scholarly publishing. They have continued to publish annual updates on their progress to implement and sustain change for the past 3 years with the latest update coming in 2023.[27,29]

AACAP Committees

AACAP has 61 committees that represent the breadth and depth of every area of child and adolescent psychiatry. These committees represent the field and are an opportunity to increase DEI initiatives. For example, in 2022, AACAP committee year-end reports indicated only 17% out of a total of 54 committees reported efforts in diversifying the workforce and professional development. Twenty-six percent reported making national partnerships and linkages to organizations dedicated to DEI (**Fig. 2**).

Given the importance of diversifying the workforce and the strong need for DEI within the AACAP organization, it is important to recognize that this must include

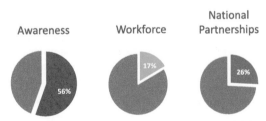

Fig. 2. Analysis of percentage of AACAP committees reporting activities promoting Awareness, Workforce and Professional Development, and National Partnerships and Linkages in the 2022 year-end reports.

changes on an organizational level. Structural changes in the form of policies must be implemented to create an environment that retains and advance the needs of a diverse workforce. As an organization that promotes the healthy development of children, adolescents, and families through advocacy, education, and research, AACAP is particularly well positioned to develop and deliver programs that support the professional development of the mental health workforce.

As part of the DEI council fellowship project, we developed methods to track, over longitudinal engagement in the priorities to measure change, which include using midyear and year-end reports, executive reports, and discussions with council leadership. For instance, the 2023 midyear report featured 2 questions related to DEI: *"(1) Has your committee engaged in any efforts related to diversity, equity, or inclusion (DEI)? (2) Has your committee updated it's charge to include DEI? Yes or No. If so, please explain?"* The qualitative analysis used content analysis methods, which were a hybrid between deductive and inductive descriptive coding. First, we analyzed all reported DEI-related activities across AACAP committees. Then, in order to understand potential areas for enhanced involvement, we evaluated committee involvement across 3 of the main priority areas: awareness, workforce diversity, and national linkages.

A total of 54 committees were consequently evaluated, along with a total of 160 midyear and year-end reports from 2021 to 2023. The analysis showed that the majority of AACAP's committees were involved in some DEI-related activities in at least one of the priority areas (**Fig. 3**). Additionally, results suggest an increase in reported activities in priority areas of awareness and workforce diversity initiatives from 2021 to 2023. Results suggest that 38% of committees have updated their charge to include DEI, an important part of the CAPture belonging priority area 5 of structural changes in AACAP. Qualitative analysis of committee reports also suggest that collaboration between committees was a key strategy for implementing DEI-focused activities. With regard to limitations, only reported activities could be quantified, and thus, this method likely underestimates the amount of DEI activities across AACAP committees.

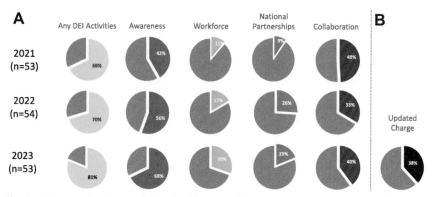

Fig. 3. Using qualitative analysis of midyear and year-end reports to monitor the involvement of committees in 3 of the main priority areas. (*A*) The results suggest increases in reported activities in priority areas of awareness and workforce diversity DEI-related activities from 2021 to 2023. (*B*) About 38% of committees updated their mission statements (charge) to include DEI. Limitations: 2023 year-end report is not yet available. Results indicated reported activities, which may underestimate the number of activities committees are engaged in.

Program Committee and Annual Meeting

The Program Committee and Meetings Department leadership are responsible for creating the experience for AACAP members at the annual gathering for AACAP. This is often an important opportunity to highlight the AACAP priorities, provide leadership and professional development opportunities, as well as reflect the direction of the organization.

Sponsorship by the Diversity and Culture Committee is one indicator of a submission's commitment to DEI at the Annual Meeting. However, many other committee submissions may also focus on DEI without sponsorship by the Diversity and Culture Committee, and so the overall number of presentations focused on DEI may be underestimated. However, when we examined the number of Diversity and Culture Committee cosponsorships for presentations accepted for the Annual Meeting during the past 4 years, it has increased overall. In 2020, there were 20 accepted submissions, and this increased to 25 in 2021 and 30 in 2022. The heightened focus on DEI-accepted submissions provides AACAP's membership with enhanced opportunities for discourse on DEI across many different areas of child and adolescent psychiatry.

In order to investigate demographic characteristics and assess for potential bias in the submission and acceptance process of the 2021 and 2022 AACAP Annual Meetings, the Program Committee analyzed submission and acceptance rates stratified by self-reported race, ethnicity, and gender. Overall, the results showed that the 2022 Annual Meeting submissions were representative of AACAP membership with an improvement from the 2021 results. In the previous year, 2021, there was a weak trend for lower Asian and Latinx/Hispanic submissions based on race and ethnicity. In 2022, there were no overall differences in submission versus acceptance rates by race, ethnicity, and gender across the Symposia and Clinical Perspectives. In 2021 and 2022, we observed weak trends, indicating lower submission versus acceptance rates for Symposia in those with Asian backgrounds and lower submission versus acceptance rates for Clinical Perspectives and Symposia among Hispanic/Latinx individuals compared with non-Hispanic White peers. Of note, symposia require more research data incorporated into the submission compared with Clinical Perspectives. These results suggest that although there have been no major differences in race, ethnicity, and gender in submissions and acceptances, we should continue monitoring AACAP's submissions and acceptance data for potential demographic disparities. Ultimately, these findings highlight the importance of ongoing efforts by AACAP to diversify the child and adolescent psychiatry physician workforce, bolster mentorship, and work toward improving representation of minoritized scholars in AACAP.

In addition to the Annual Meeting, AACAP's Clinical Essentials Committee, has developed an online CME learning portal, entitled Pathways, to provide learning and professional development throughout the year. Two new modules: "Advancing Anti-Racism and Social Justice Action," and "Racism, Injustice, and Inequities," were introduced.

AACAP Assembly of Regional Organizations

Regional organizations are the grassroots level components of AACAP that are responsible for local support of members, addressing statewide issues, advocacy, and collaborations. The Assembly is composed of delegates from all 58 member regional organizations. There are elected Assembly officers who serve an executive function and represent the regional organizations within the AACAP governing Council board. The Assembly Executive Committee comprises a Chair and 6 members with trends toward diverse representation. In 2021, the Chair was BIPOC and the executive committee was 71% BIPOC and 71% women. In 2022, the Chair was a woman and

BIPOC and the executive committee was 57% BIPOC and 71% women and 86% POC.

During the past 3 years, regional organizations are required to send reports to AACAP leadership before the biannual Assembly meetings. In 2021 and 2022, 13% of the reports submitted before the meetings identified specific DEI initiatives or activities (eg, creating a DEI committee, DEI programming at the annual conference). In 2023, a new section of the report specifically requested identification of any DEI program or activities. Since this was added, we observed a 33% increase in reports of DEI programming, with 46% of regional organizations in the first half of 2023 responding so far. This percentage may increase because there is another report reflecting the second half of 2023. However, this already represents an increase during the past few years. A likely factor may include the importance of intentionally requesting DEI information. This will enable AACAP to demonstrate any change over time as a target priority. Importantly, having national DEI priorities manifest in local articles is a critical part of ensuring that our DEI goals are met.

Department of Government Affairs

AACAP has developed policy priorities for the Department of Government Affairs to take actions to drive federal and state advocacy efforts. One of the 3 priorities highlighted DEI issues for the first time. In both 2022 and 2023, AACAP prioritized improving equity in access to child and adolescent psychiatry specifically to ensure that pediatric mental health care systems addressed the needs of racial and ethnic minoritized youth, families, and communities. The specific legislation highlighted during the 2022 and 2023 AACAP Legislative conferences promoted the Pursuing Equity in Mental Health Act, targeted at building a more diverse mental health workforce and increasing DEI competencies across mental health interventions. In 2023, AACAP promoted the Conrad State 30 Physician Access Reauthorization Act to increase diversity among the physician workforce, leveraging the national platform of the Legislative conference to take action in coalition with youth and families. AACAP also issued 9 Presidential statements highlighting DEI issues in 2022/2023 and endorsed 9 House and Senate bills supporting DEI in mental health-care legislation. Almost half of the attendees to the Legislative Conference have been trainees in both 2022 and 2023. Furthermore, out of the 86 trainees who attended the Legislative Conference in 2023, 47% were BIPOC and even more annually through monthly advocacy efforts, ensuring that diverse trainees have opportunities to have their values reflected in the AACAP actions.

Membership

As an organization, an important component of achieving AACAP's DEI goals has been to implement a more standardized process of collecting racial, ethnic, gender, and other demographic identification to reflect the membership and DEI dimensions. Preliminary demographic findings for 2023 are shown in **Table 2** but improved data collection methods are needed given 24% missing race/ethnicity data. The Joint Commitment for Action on Inclusion and Diversity in Publishing, a consortium of more than 50 organizations representing more than 15,000 journals was used to help inform this process.[32] Improving the data will help the organization have more meaningful information. AACAP has worked toward establishing, standardizing, and implementing a common tool to help capture the identifying data across the different components of AACAP. This will help the organization develop a method of reviewing DEI data across the organization.

Based on these analyses, we found evidence that implementation of AACAP's strategic plan to enhance the diversity of the child psychiatry and child mental health workforce across all mission areas has been successful in increasing DEI activities across committees and the priority areas of awareness, advocacy, and workforce and professional development. Options for improvement in the future include an increased focus on developing national partnerships and linkages with DEI-focused organizations. In addition, continued collaboration across AACAP committees may be beneficial for continued increases in DEI-related progress. Finally, improved record keeping of DEI-related activities will ensure more complete and fruitful analysis in the future.

SUMMARY

In summary, this article has discussed AACAP's strategic plan for diversifying the child and adolescent psychiatry workforce. Leadership prioritization of DEI priorities is key to achieving success and transformation. The strategic plan had 3 pillars: promoting DEI across all mission areas, creating a pipeline of child and adolescent psychiatrists, and monitoring DEI activities and progress on an organizational level. With regard to promoting DEI across all mission areas, this involved developing a taskforce who developed a 5-point action plan, which was championed by the president's initiative, CAPture Belonging. This action plan involved creating awareness, enhancing advocacy, building workforce and pipelines, strengthening national partnerships, and ensuring sustainability through governing documents and principles. Creating a pipeline of child and adolescent psychiatrists was addressed by creating a community of belonging while investing in new leadership fellowships, expansion of mentorship, enhancement of antiracist scholarly journal review processes, and increasing transparency and opportunities. Grants were awarded with the focus of creating a pipeline of diverse child and adolescent psychiatrists in research and clinical care. Creating a culture where DEI is embedded within the organization's governing principles and actions is important to sustainability. All components of AACAP need to reflect an ongoing commitment to DEI framework and the collective goal of creating a community of belonging. Methods will continue to be developed and refined to best measure change over time. Currently, the monitoring of these efforts was accomplished through quantitative and qualitative analysis of 160 committee reports, 71 regional organization reports, executive annual reports, 2 legislative conferences, and different initiatives during 3 years. Results indicate evidence of successful implementation of AACAP's strategic plan for advancing DEI priorities and diversifying the workforce in child and adolescent psychiatry. Developing an updated demographic identification tool across all of the AACAP components will be important to help measure sustained progress.

CLINICS CARE POINTS

- Promoting DEI goals across AACAP's mission areas required embedding DEI initiatives into the organization on a structural level.
- Support for a pipeline of child and adolescent psychiatrists involved enhancing leadership opportunities, expansion of mentorship, and promoting diversity in scholarly activities.
- Monitoring DEI activities at an organizational level is important to sustain progress toward goals.

ACKNOWLEDGEMENTS

We have no acknowledgements.

DISCLOSURE

T.R. Brown, W.Y.K. Ng, and T.D. Benton declare no financial conflicts of interest. There was no funding for this article.

REFERENCES

1. Lee PC, Flores JM, Adams A, et al. Who we are today: a national survey of diversity among psychiatry program directors. Acad Psychiatry 2021;45(1):43–8.
2. Redford G. AAMC releases strategic plan to respond to rapidly changing health care landscape. AAMC 2020. Available at: https://www.aamc.org/news/aamc-releases-strategic-plan-respond-rapidly-changing-health-care-landscape. Accessed July 8, 2023.
3. Office of the Surgeon General (US). Mental health: a report of the surgeon general. Dept. Of health and human services, U.S. Public health service. For sale by the Supt. of Docs.; 1999.
4. Office of the Surgeon General (US), Center for Mental Health Services (US), National Institute of Mental Health (US). Mental health: culture, race, and ethnicity: a supplement to mental health: a report of the surgeon general. (US): Substance Abuse and Mental Health Services Administration; 2001. Available at: http://www.ncbi.nlm.nih.gov/books/NBK44243/. Accessed August 29, 2023.
5. Meghani SH, Brooks JM, Gipson-Jones T, et al. Patient–provider race-concordance: does it matter in improving minority patients' health outcomes? Ethn Health 2009;14(1):107–30.
6. Santiago CD, Miranda J. Progress in improving mental health services for racial-ethnic minority groups: a ten-year perspective. PS 2014;65(2):180–5.
7. Baah FO, Teitelman AM, Riegel B. Marginalization: conceptualizing patient vulnerabilities in the framework of social determinants of health – an integrative review. Nurs Inq 2019;26(1):e12268.
8. Paradies Y, Ben J, Denson N, et al. Racism as a determinant of health: a systematic review and meta-analysis. PLoS One 2015;10(9):e0138511.
9. Brown TR, Xu KY, Glowinski AL. Cognitive behavioral therapy and the implementation of antiracism. JAMA Psychiatr 2021;78(8):819–20.
10. Hall WJ, Chapman MV, Lee KM, et al. Implicit racial/ethnic bias among health care professionals and its influence on health care outcomes: a systematic review. Am J Publ Health 2015;105(12):e60–76.
11. Jones CP. Levels of racism: a theoretic framework and a gardener's tale. Am J Publ Health 2000;90(8):1212–5.
12. Campbell KM, Corral I, Infante Linares JL, et al. Projected estimates of african american medical graduates of closed historically black medical schools. JAMA Netw Open 2020;3(8):e2015220.
13. Laws T. How should we respond to racist legacies in health professions education originating in the flexner report? AMA Journal of Ethics 2021;23(3):271–5.
14. Avakame EF, October TW, Dixon GL. Antiracism in academic medicine: fixing the leak in the pipeline of black physicians. ATS Scholar 2021;2(2):193–201.
15. Widge AS, Jordan A, Kraguljac NV, et al. Structural racism in psychiatric research careers: eradicating barriers to a more diverse workforce. Am J Psychiatry 2023; 180(9):645–59.
16. HHS Office of Population Affairs. America's Diverse Adolescents | HHS Office of Population Affairs. Published 2019. Available at: https://opa.hhs.gov/adolescent-health/adolescent-health-facts/americas-diverse-adolescents. Accessed August 29, 2023.

17. AAMC. Diversity in medicine: facts and Figures 2019. AAMC; 2019. Available at: https://www.aamc.org/data-reports/workforce/report/diversity-medicine-facts-and-figures-2019. Accessed August 27, 2023.
18. AAMC. Number of people per active physician by specialty, 2021. AAMC; 2021. Available at: https://www.aamc.org/data-reports/workforce/data/number-people-active-physician-specialty-2021. Accessed August 27, 2023.
19. AAMC. Percentage change in the number of active physicians by specialty, 2016-2021. AAMC; 2021. Available at: https://www.aamc.org/data-reports/workforce/data/percentage-change-number-active-physicians-specialty-2016-2021. Accessed August 27, 2023.
20. AAMC. ACGME Residents and Fellows by Sex and Specialty, 2021. AAMC. Available at: https://www.aamc.org/data-reports/workforce/data/acgme-residents-fellows-sex-and-specialty-2021. Accessed August 28, 2023.
21. AAMC. Percentage Change in Number of First-Year ACGME Residents and Fellows by Specialty, 2016-2021. AAMC. Available at: https://www.aamc.org/data-reports/workforce/data/percentage-change-first-year-acgme-residents-fellows-specialty-2016-2021. Accessed August 28, 2023.
22. AAMC. Diversity increases at medical schools in 2022. AAMC; 2022. Available at: https://www.aamc.org/news/press-releases/diversity-increases-medical-schools-2022. Accessed August 27, 2023.
23. Rubin R. How the SCOTUS affirmative action ruling could affect medical schools and health care. JAMA 2023;330(6):492–4.
24. Schmidt H, Gostin LO, Williams MA. The Supreme court's rulings on race neutrality threaten progress in medicine and health. JAMA 2023. https://doi.org/10.1001/jama.2023.13749.
25. AACAP. Anti Racism Resource Library. Available at: https://www.aacap.org/AACAP/Families_Youth/Resource_Libraries/Anti-Racism_Resource_Library/AACAP/Families_and_Youth/Resource_Libraries/Racism_Resource_Library.aspx?hkey=78228df4-6ab6-4ed6-8757-4f412d8921e4. Accessed September 12, 2023.
26. AACAP. Cultural Diversity Resource Center. Available at: https://www.aacap.org/aacap/Families_and_Youth/Resource_Centers/Cultural_Diversity_Resource_Center/Home.aspx. Accessed September 12, 2023.
27. Novins DK, Althoff RR, Cortese S, et al. Editors' note: first annual report regarding JAACAP's antiracist journey. J Am Acad Child Adolesc Psychiatr 2021;60(12):1448–51.
28. AACAP. Medical Students. Available at: https://www.aacap.org/AACAP/Your_Career/AACAP/Medical_Students_and_Residents/Medical_Students/Home.aspx. Accessed September 12, 2023.
29. Novins DK, Althoff RR, Cortese S, et al. Our vision: an antiracist journal. J Am Acad Child Adolesc Psychiatr 2020;59(10):1105–6.
30. Novins DK, Althoff RR, Cortese S, et al. Editors' note: second annual report regarding JAACAP's antiracist journey. J Am Acad Child Adolesc Psychiatr 2022;61(12):1405–10.
31. NIH. NIH Commitment to Diversity | Diversity in Extramural Programs. Available at: https://extramural-diversity.nih.gov/building-participation/commitment-across-nih. Accessed August 29, 2023.
32. Royal Society of Chemistry. Diversity data collection in scholarly publishing. Royal Society of Chemistry; 2022. Available at: https://www.rsc.org/policy-evidence-campaigns/inclusion-diversity/joint-commitment-for-action-inclusion-and-diversity-in-publishing/diversity-data-collection-in-scholarly-publishing/. Accessed August 27, 2023.

33. AAMC. 2022 Physician Specialty Data Report Tables 1.10a-1.10h. AAMC. Available at: https://www.aamc.org/data-reports/data/2022-physician-specialty-data-report-executive-summary. Accessed August 28, 2023.
34. AAMC. Table B5. Number of active MD residents, by race/ethnicity (alone or in combination) and GME specialty. AAMC; 2021. Available at: https://www.aamc.org/data-reports/students-residents/data/report-residents/2022/table-b5-md-residents-race-ethnicity-and-specialty. Accessed August 27, 2023.
35. AAMC. Table A-14.3: Race/Ethnicity Responses (Alone and In Combination) of Matriculants to U.S. MD-Granting Medical Schools, 2018-2019 through 2022-2023. Published 2023. Accessed August 27, 2023. https://www.aamc.org/media/8826/download?attachment.

Moving?

Make sure your subscription moves with you!

To notify us of your new address, find your **Clinics Account Number** (located on your mailing label above your name), and contact customer service at:

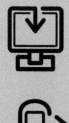

Email: journalscustomerservice-usa@elsevier.com

800-654-2452 (subscribers in the U.S. & Canada)
314-447-8871 (subscribers outside of the U.S. & Canada)

Fax number: 314-447-8029

Elsevier Health Sciences Division
Subscription Customer Service
3251 Riverport Lane
Maryland Heights, MO 63043

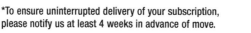

Printed and bound by CPI Group (UK) Ltd, Croydon, CR0 4YY

03/10/2024

01040466-0008